HEALTH CARE, ENTITLEMENT, AND CITIZENSHIP

Access to universal health care has become a symbol of Canadian national identity. It is also one of the most contentious and politically charged issues in the field of public policy in Canada. In this study, Candace Johnson Redden examines the theoretical dimensions of citizenship and rights in Canada as they intersect with health care politics. She offers possible answers to questions concerning the philosophical and political meanings of the right to health care in advanced industrial societies, the equitable distribution of health care resources in those societies, and the effects of globalization and fractured patterns of citizenship on discussions of entitlement, universal human rights, and bioethics.

Redden proposes that recent trends in citizenship development will require a health care system that is capable of recognizing the different citizenships across Canada, flexible enough to accommodate many different citizenship claims, and consequently able to facilitate interaction between communities and governments. This interdisciplinary study examines epidemiological, technological, and political patterns, and will appeal to anyone interested in Canadian politics, public policy, citizenship, and health care.

CANDACE JOHNSON REDDEN is an Assistant Professor in the Department of Community Health Sciences at Brock University.

The Institute of Public Administration of Canada
Series in Public Management and Governance

Editor: Peter Aucoin

This series is sponsored by the Institute of Public Administration of Canada as part of its commitment to encourage research on issues in Canadian public administration, public sector management, and public policy. It also seeks to foster wider knowledge and understanding among practioners, academics, and the general public.

Networks of Knowledge: Collaborative Innovation in International Learning
Janice Stein, Richard Stren, Joy Fitzgibbon, and Melissa MacLean

The National Research Council in the Innovative Policy Era: Changing Hierarchies, Networks, and Markets
G. Bruce Doern and Richard Levesque

Beyond Service: State Workers, Public Policy, and the Prospects for Democratic Administration
Greg McElligott

Policy-Making by Administrative Tribunal: How the Ontario Municipal Board Has Developed and Applied Land Use Planning Policy
John G. Chipman

Health Care, Entitlement, and Citizenship
Candace Johnson Redden

CANDACE JOHNSON REDDEN

Health Care, Entitlement, and Citizenship

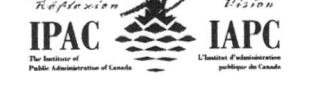

UNIVERSITY OF TORONTO PRESS
Toronto Buffalo London

© University of Toronto Press Incorporated 2002
Toronto Buffalo London
Printed in Canada

ISBN 0-8020-3626-0 (cloth)
ISBN 0-8020-8466-4 (paper)

Printed on acid-free paper

National Library of Canada Cataloguing in Publication

Redden, Candace Johnson
  Health care, entitlement and citizenship / Candace Johnson Redden.

(The Institute of Public Administration of Canada series in public
management and governance)
Includes bibliographical references and index.
ISBN 0-8020-3626-0 (bound)   ISBN 0-8020-8466-4 (pbk.)

1. Right to health care – Canada.   2. Medical policy – Canada.
3. Citizenship – Canada.   I. Institute of Public Administration of
Canada.   II. Title.   III. Series: Institute of Public Administration of
Canada series in public management and governance.

RA395.C3R435 2002   362.1'0971   C2002-901516-2

This book has been published with the help of a grant from the Humanities
and Social Sciences Federation of Canada, using funds provided by the
Social Sciences and Humanities Research Council of Canada.

University of Toronto Press acknowledges the financial assistance to its
publishing program of the Canada Council for the Arts and the Ontario Arts
Council.

University of Toronto Press acknowledges the financial support for its
publishing activities of the Government of Canada through the Book
Publishing Industry Development Program (BPIDP).

Contents

Acknowledgments

The initial idea for this work was inspired while I was an undergraduate student at the University of Toronto. In a course on comparative public administration, Professor David Wolfe introduced me to the literature on social rights and citizenship. And Professors Alkis Kontos and Ronald Beiner demonstrated the power and mystique of political philosophy. I am certain that none of these professors remembers me, but they had an impact on me just the same. Most of the scholarly work I have done since then has been an effort to reconcile social policy and philosophical perspectives.

The first incarnation of this project was my doctoral dissertation, written at Dalhousie University. I would like to thank Peter Aucoin and Lawrence Nestman for serving on my dissertation committee. Their advice and encouragement are much appreciated. Pat Armstrong was the external examiner for the thesis. Her involvement was generous. Her supportive and constructive comments were indispensable and helped to shape the final version of the project. I would like to thank Dalhousie University for financial assistance throughout the program. Thanks also to two incredible colleagues, Allison Young and Anna Lanoszka. On many occasions they helped me to think through tedious and complex (not to mention tiresome) arguments. Allison taught me about the importance of strategy and relentless social analysis and kept me sane with marathon telephone conversations and trips to New York. And Anna kept me smiling with 'Adult Pepsi,' Salman Rushdie, and long lunches.

While I was conducting research for this book I had the opportunity to interview a number of people in Nova Scotia and Saskatchewan. I am grateful to all who shared their information and insights. In particular, I would like to thank Ken Dueck for the time that he spent acquainting me with the dynamics of health politics and system reform in Saskatchewan.

The final stages of research and writing were completed while I was a Visiting Assistant Professor at American University in Washington, DC. I owe a huge debt of gratitude to Karen O'Connor for everything, including but not limited to the following: befriending me, giving me a job, introducing me to women and politics, and feminist theory research, encouraging me to publish my work, reading and commenting on various manuscripts, directing a naïve neophyte scholar through the maze of academe, and helping a reticent Canadian to meet other scholars. Thanks, Karen, for putting yourself in my corner. I couldn't have done any of this without you. Thanks also to several other fantastic colleagues: to David Lublin for his ideas, advice, encouragement, and friendship, and for keeping me apprised of Canadian current events. To fellow Bohemian scholar, Joe Soss, for his support and intellectual inspiration. To Bob Boucher for his much valued friendship. To Nathan Dietz for his kindness and good humour, and for his willingness to indulge in some afternoon chocolate with me. Thanks also to Sarah E. Brewer and Erin O'Brien for NEW Leadership (Sarah), The Backstreet Boys (Erin), and for listening to my lengthy job talk (twice!). I would like to acknowledge Shelby Austin, my student, teaching assistant, and good friend. Last but certainly not least, thanks to Michael Fisher for his humbling intelligence and sharp wit. I benefited from both on a regular basis.

I am very grateful to A.R. Gillis, Professor of Sociology at the University of Toronto, for supporting and encouraging me throughout all of my endeavours. It has always been comforting to know that he is only a phone call away. I would also like to acknowledge my best friend, Melanie Gillis. Her support and love are unfailing and indispensable.

Thanks are also in order for John Hay, Chair of the Department of Community Health Sciences at Brock University, for allowing me time to complete this project before taking up my new position in that department.

At University of Toronto Press, I would like to thank Virgil Duff. I am grateful to the anonymous readers who reviewed the manuscript. Thanks also to Kate Baltais, who copyedited the manuscript, and Mary Newberry for preparing the index.

Earlier versions of some chapters, or parts of chapters, have appeared in the *Canadian Journal of Political Science*, the *Journal of Health Politics, Policy, and Law,* and in the Institute of Intergovernmental Relations (Queen's University) Working Paper Series.

Special thanks are owed to my parents, Linda and Don Johnson, and my brother, Tyson Johnson, for their love and assistance. I dedicate this book to them.

HEALTH CARE, ENTITLEMENT, AND CITIZENSHIP

1

Introduction

Debates concerning health care in Canada and the United States have reached a significant juncture. There is regular cross-border dialogue and comparison in this policy field, and approaches to reform emanating from historically disparate paths in each country seem to be converging. Universality and privatization both seem to be untenable. In the United States, the possibility of universal access to health care services is addressed in ambitious, idealistic, and contradictory ways, with increasing alarm and frustration. In Canada, universal health care is being eroded by rising levels of private sector involvement in both the insurance and delivery of health care services; this has provoked defensive responses from citizens, often in the form of rights claims for entrenched patterns of entitlement.

Do citizens really have a right to health care? If they do, does that right provide much, if any, philosophical or political resistance to unwanted changes in the health care system? In this book, I draw on political theory and public policy literatures to address one deceptively simple question: How has the idea of the right to health care evolved in Canada, and what does it mean now, at the beginning of the twenty-first century? The answer to this question is important. It will reveal something about what we may anticipate for patterns of health service distribution and something about the substance of citizenship.

The relevance of health care to debates concerning citizenship has been consistently overlooked by both political theorists and health policy scholars, yet the relationship is an important one. Although it can be argued that the right to health care does not count as a natural right, namely, a right carried by each human being from the state of nature into society, it is, nevertheless, clear that access to health services has a great impact on each individual's quality of life. Rights, privacy, and the autonomy of citizens constitute one side of the citizenship equation, their duties and obligations constitute the other. At face value, the exchange appears to be a straightforward transaction between the citizen and the state, one aimed at achieving some workable level of solidarity or connectedness. Debate surrounds the balance of the equation – how burdensome ought the duties be, to what extent should rights in their absolute form be protected, and how much diversity can be accommodated within structures designed to foster unity? The apparent neutrality of rights, the quintessential component of contemporary citizenship,[1] is misleading in that it often precludes a deeper probing of citizenship 'bargains.' The language of rights cannot secure a neutral political arrangement, nor can it fully explain the mercurial dynamics of citizenship. Of course, this observation is not novel, and does not yet fully explain how health care is linked to conceptual and substantive discussions of citizenship.

Canada's current constitutional and citizenship arrangements include a substantial commitment to multiculturalism. What it means to be a Canadian is multifarious. The Canadian identity is composed of many different identities, and this is celebrated, not lamented. Formal recognition of diversity among the populace makes Canada unique. Although many aspects of the Canadian citizenship experience are shared, it is by no means imperative that all Canadians have identical social, political, and cultural identities. To the contrary, as a country Canada has decided that its national identity is enriched by diversity and heterogeneity.

The balance between sameness, consistency, and equality for the sake of unity and social cohesion, on the one hand, and recognition and respect of cultural and ethnic diversity, on the other, has been a historical challenge for Canada. The Quebec Act of 1774 guaranteed for Quebec constitutional respect for difference, and it set the precedent for Quebec's asymmetrical position within the Canadian federation. This asymmetry was maintained until 1982 and, to some extent, is still maintained. The Canadian Charter of Rights and Freedoms revisioned and recreated the Canadian constitutional bargain so that (1) all individuals were granted rights that, for the most part, could not be altered by governments; and (2) rights were granted to groups based on culture, ethnicity, and gender. The first diluted Quebec's claim for difference. Individual Canadians acquired a new status that might not allow an alternate vision of citizenship in Quebec. The second frustrated Quebec's claim for distinctness by allowing other groups the same claim.

Health care is an important component of Canadian citizenship and identity, perhaps tantamount to culture. The recognition of rights based on culture has transformed citizenship, and has reinforced respect for both individuals and groups. Health care has been, and should be, similarly transformed. The Canada Health Act (1984) establishes conditions for the federal disbursement of transfer payments to the provinces and guarantees, in general terms, levels of service and access for individual Canadians. As will be explained in the chapters that follow, the claim for health care as a right is increasingly legalistic and individualistic. In part, this is the legacy of the Canada Health Act and the Charter of Rights and Freedoms, which departed from earlier patterns of entitlement. 'The right to health care' is ingrained with collectivist thought currently threatened by reform efforts. It is the communal component that needs further consideration and investigation. If the pattern for Canadian citizenship as it relates to policy for multiculturalism is one that tries to reconcile equality and difference, unity and diversity, then would the same pattern or approach make sense for health care? Claiming health care as a right may actually constrain necessary change in the health care system, while differentiated citizenship may provide a model for new patterns of access and entitlement to health care services.

Differentiated Citizenship and Multiculturalism

Throughout the 1990s there was much scholarly debate engaged-in by political scientists, theorists, and philosophers over the merits of granting 'recognition' for 'difference' to cultural minorities through group rights. Proponents of recognition include Iris Marion Young, Will Kymlicka, Charles Taylor, Michael Sandel, and James Tully.[2] They effectively defend recognition in theoretical debates concerning rights, citizenship, and the 'Good Society,' and at the same time they provide new ways to think about urgent political matters. Although there is great variation in the details of their arguments, all have a common theme: 'On this view [of differentiated citizenship], members of certain groups would be incorporated into the political community not only as individuals but also through the group, and their rights would depend, in part, on their group membership.'[3] The merits of such an approach, in both philosophical and pragmatic political terms, have been widely disputed. However, the possibility of applying the approach to health care debates has not been considered.

In Canada, there are two poles of discussion concerning health care: defence of the existing, if imperfect, universal arrangements, and promotion of increased privatization of health services. In the highly ideological health care debate in the United States, health care reformers seem to approach the policy issue with either fruitless, piecemeal changes, or catastrophic, all-or-nothing reasoning.

The need for new approaches to health care policy in Canada, and in other countries, is pressing and real. One position, explored in this book, submits that a differentiated approach to recognizing the needs of communities might best equalize the substance of citizenship by providing particular information about the identities of relevant groups, thus establishing a broader context for health care debates. The first daunting step entails the classification of identifiable communities as bases for providing appropriate health care services and resources. Certainly, there will be some overlap of cultural minorities and communities relevant to health care, such as Native persons and women, but in other cases there would be new categories of entitlement to health services. These new categories would include citizen-patients with HIV/AIDS and the elderly who already have access to additional goods as members of those communities. However, it is becoming increasingly clear that a more deliberate and definitive approach is needed to carving out new patterns of access to health care in Canada.

Rights and Compensation

Approaches that achieve social cohesion and at the same time respect difference contribute a political dimension to the arguments of Richard Wilkinson, Paul Farmer, and Robert G. Evans, Morris Barer, and Theodore Marmor.[4] The prevailing epidemiological consensus is that there is an underlying risk pattern for health and disease that is socially determined. In their thorough investigation, Evans, Barer, and Marmor conclude that even when factors such as lifestyle (levels of exercise, dietary habits, alcohol consumption, and tobacco use) and stress level (based on job security, income sufficient to meet needs, proportion of disposable income, and relative happiness in life) are controlled, poorer people are still less healthy.[5] This profound sociological fact escapes reliable medical explanation. It is most succinctly and clearly put by Sophie Tucker: 'I've been poor, and I've been rich. Rich is better.'[6]

Richard Wilkinson states that 'it is now clear that the scale of income differences in a society is one of the most powerful determinants of health standards in different countries, and that it influences health through its impact on social cohesion.'[7] Adding to this finding, Paul Farmer submits that identity politics is self-serving, further disruptive of social cohesion, and therefore a threat to the health of a population.[8] However, Farmer fails to recognize the impossibility, in political terms, of ignoring differences based on identity in multicultural, multi-ethnic states.

It is socially and medically responsible to identify the effects of social class and relative income disparity on health. It is, however, politically naïve to suggest that a social rights or welfare state approach will remedy inequality, and thereby improve the health of everyone in the society. Social cohesion will not be achieved solely through mechanisms designed to flatten income distributions. In Canada and the United States, measures to counteract the polarization of the wealthy and the poor are vital in fostering greater social cohesion and improving the health of all citizens. It is also imperative in both of these multicultural, multi-ethnic countries that identity rights are recognized as a means to locate and remedy patterns of inequality. To achieve greater cohesion through the recognition of difference, it is necessary to positively identify communities, and then determine their patterns of access and entitlement to health care services as a matter of citizenship.

Identity and Social Cohesion: Unity from Difference?

Approaches that might bridge the gap between social cohesion and difference, or foster unity from difference, offer grounds for a complex discussion. As argued by leading citizenship theorists, such as Kymlicka and Young, social cohesion in large, multicultural, multi-ethnic states can best be achieved through the recognition of differentiated citizenship claims. The goal of unity does not entail glossing over persistent and structural inequalities, but calling them out. Further, these theorists argue that the state should not try to remain neutral in face of social inequalities and ethical preferences, which might reflect and exacerbate those inequalities, but it should begin to determine what differences, discounted in the past, should be valued, and which groups – because this discounting has resulted in marginalization – are entitled to compensation.

Young's 1990 work on identity politics is still one of the most important points of departure for debates in this area. Through positive respect for difference, valuing and recognizing various identities rather than tolerating them, the promise of citizenship can be realized.[9] The problems of such an approach are apparent. It will not be easy to identify candidates for recognition because, presumably, all people have the potential for some claim for compensation.[10] Even if such candidates could be identified, their 'difference' might have a divisive effect, which is antithetical to citizenship's commitment to unity and cohesion.

These problems, endemic to debates concerning multiculturalism, are less burdensome for health care debates. The impossibility of separating authentic from strategic identity does not confound theories of identity and differentiated citizenship for health politics. The groups suggested as candidates for compensation in future health policy, HIV/AIDS patients, and the elderly, for instance, have identities insofar as they are socially constructed. There is nothing authentic to be recognized in either group, in the way that it might be recognized in cultural and ethnic groups. Recognition is to serve a specifically practical and not an engulfing purpose. Universality in health care will be achieved by asking who suffers the greatest inequality in the current system and by delivering services and benefits accordingly.

The postwar orthodoxy of social rights, in the form of universal entitlements for health insurance, has been seriously and, to some extent, successfully challenged by the multiculturalists.[11] Does it make sense, then, for health policy scholars and practitioners to continue to blindly defend universal entitlements? Clearly, there are advantages to maintaining the universal health care system in Canada. Canadian health care is a source of pride for citizens, and the benefits secured through the system guarantee a great measure of security, stability, and even identity.

The Canadian system serves as a model around the globe, and proves Canada's social policy superiority in North America. Nevertheless, Canadian reformers cannot, and should not, rest on their laurels. The health care system faces a growing number of challenges that might not be resolved unless postwar commitments to universality are reconceived. It is desirable, for both practical and symbolic reasons, to maintain commitments to universality; yet, it may be the case that a fair and just distribution of health care might not translate as a strictly equal distribution. Different people and groups of people will need to use health care resources in varying ways. Efforts at reform should try to reflect the diversity of these needs, not dissolve them into existing commitments to universality. Health care may be viewed as intersectional. Indeed, health status overlaps with cultural and social identities. Understanding the ways in which environment, culture, and society affect health is a distinct and unavoidable challenge for all of us who are concerned about the progress of social policy.

Claims for cultural diversity are based, in some cases, on notions of authenticity. There is something authentic, that is, genuine and true, and therefore valuable and deserving of respect, in being Aboriginal or Québécois. In addition, there is some compensation owed members of these groups for historical wrongs and continued marginalization. Groups privileged by virtue of their difference are not candidates for recognition. Thus, respect for diversity celebrates authenticity, while at the same time it addresses inequality. Groups marginalized because their cultural, ethnic, or social identity is devalued, experience additional, predictable forms of social inequality including differences in health care status and in access to health care services.

A Note on Method

The conceptual framework for this project is an intersection of rights theory (including social rights discourse, which has its roots in sociology) and citizenship theory. As such, this book contributes to ongoing theoretical debates concerning the value and substance of rights and their utility in mediating the citizen–state relationship. The debate concerning the value of absolute rights relative to various conceptions of the 'good society' is directly relevant to health care politics. The degree to which Canadians determine their own national identity in contradistinction to the perceived ruthless rights orientation of U.S. society will affect the possibilities for health care reform in Canada.

The book also addresses health care as a public policy issue. Important works in the fields of political science, sociology, and epidemiology are analysed and synthesized, and set in the context of the theoretical discussion. For example, recent developments in the province of Alberta concerning overnight stays in private clinics are a challenge to the prevailing normative constitution of Canadian society, as well as the authority of the federal government in enforcing provincial compliance with the Canada Health Act. Central to reform debates are governments' fiscal restraint measures in competition with media coverage of hopelessly long emergency room waits, and the alarming lack of resources available to hospitals, physicians, and other caregivers. All indications are that Canadians' entitlements to health care are on a collision course with governments' ability to fund services.

Outline

As governments devise health care reform strategies to respond to the changing dynamics of budgeting, federalism, and health, citizens resist changes to what they perceive to be their social rights of citizenship. Such resistance is beneficial in that it serves to protect entitlement and secure health care as a symbol of national identity. However, the right to health care has been defended categorically as an infungible, sustainable element of the state–society relationship in spite of the evolutionary nature of social citizenship. Furthermore, the meaning of 'the right to health care' has never really been determined. What do citizens mean when they say that they have the right to health care? Are they claiming collective entitlement, or individual moral property? Chapter 2 offers a critical examination of T.H. Marshall's social rights thesis[12] and sets the stage for the main argument of the book. In Chapter 3, I begin the central argument by demonstrating that the right to health care has changed significantly over the past fifty years in response to a variety of forces, many pulling in the same direction. This argument will serve to examine two major problems with the social rights thesis; Marshall's analysis pertains directly to Britain, and addresses issues of education and poverty, which necessitate modifications to fully understand the importance and effect of the social rights thesis in different geographic contexts and in regard to health care (these problems are also addressed obliquely throughout the work). More specifically, Chapter 3 addresses one of the most troubling aspects of contemporary defences of Marshall's analysis: there remains a unidimensional account of inequality.

By the end of Chapter 4, it will be clear that the right to health care in Canada is most accurately conceived as a second-order human right, reliant on ought statements rather than on the precepts of natural law. As such, the right to health care is fluid, and changing, as citizenship develops beyond the social rights stage. Citizenship development is pushed by changes in constitutional arrangements, public management practices, and corresponding citizen expectations. Paradoxically, as expectations advance, they also stay the same. This is to say that citizens' expectations rise incrementally; new expectations build on, rather than replace, previously held and institutionalized expectations. The result is policy stasis.

In Chapter 5, I argue that social rights stasis is reinforced by the dynamics of budgeting, the politics of federalism, and citizens' fear of privatization. Social rights made more sense in the context of Keynesianism (domestic commitments to balancing the economy through counter-cyclical economic management), 'relaxed scarcity,'[13] and post–Second World War nationalism, and is somewhat outmoded in budgeting environments marked by increasing numbers of competitive claims. The goal of governance since the 1990s has become respecting the diversity of these claims, not dissolving them into withering commitments to universality.

Chapter 6 argues that policy stasis is problematic because of its consequences for health. The shift in main causes of death from communicable to non-communicable diseases (the epidemiological transition), requires a new blend of individual responsibility-taking and collective entitlement, as well as more flexible approaches to the delivery of health care services. Defences of social rights, as originally formulated, reinforce the medical model at the same time that they recognize the need for change. The argument of Chapter 6 serves to complement that of the previous chapters in explaining the main causes of confusion and lack of change in the health policy field. Building on Chapter 4, Chapter 6 introduces analysis at the institutional and system levels as a means of giving substance to the conceptual component of the work and establishing a context for the following policy-specific chapter.

Chapter 7 addresses another major problem with Marshall's conception of social rights: defenders have neglected the reciprocal nature of the state–society relationship. In Chapter 7 I argue that provincial exercises in community engagement for health care decision-making might provide important opportunities for citizens to fulfil their duties of citizenship. That is, citizens can become more active in determining the ways in which health care is delivered in the context of technological advancement, alternative service provision, changing demographics and epidemiological patterns, and finite resources. The problem is that such opportunities might be undermined by social rights stasis, which perpetuates the existing welfare state model. It is argued, moreover, that there needs to be greater attention paid to the ways in which identity-based entities interact with geographically based entities. The development of community governance structures for health care, a major component of provincial health care reform packages, is considered in detail and is suggestive, if not representative, of other trends in health policy. Chapter 7 crystallizes several lines of argument and concludes that differentiated citizenship claims might be accommodated and promoted by a more fragmented and localized set of decision-making structures because citizen and community empowerment and consultation can inform policy reform and provide some balance to the power of the medical profession.

This argument is concluded in Chapter 8 with an evaluation of the development of social citizenship in Canada. The empirical evidence and theoretical arguments presented indicate that Canada is entering a fourth stage of citizenship development. Of course, not all problems of the third stage were solved, and health care as Canada's sacred trust and irresolvable social policy dilemma is not likely to be perfected in the next stage, either. But, in order that change can be effected, it is essential to understand that the social rights thesis, as popularly defended, is outmoded.

Conclusion

Throughout this book, I argue that citizenship in Canada has developed beyond social rights and towards the reconciliation of identity rights and federalism. My central questions: how have social rights become institutionalized in Canada, and what are the political implications of the institutionalization of social rights of citizenship? are relevant to, and have implications for, reform efforts in other parts of the globe. The impossibility of Canada maintaining current arrangements for its successful social policy bargain – universal health care as a component of citizenship – is a conclusion significant for social justice, national identity, and comparative public policy.

The temporal period for this analysis is approximately 1966 (the year in which public medical insurance was implemented at the national level in Canada) to the September 2000 First Ministers Conference, although much of the analysis has a broader historical context. As the universal health care system developed throughout the 1940s, 1950s, and 1960s, and as the range of available services expanded, citizens' expectations were elevated. By 1980, when retrenchment was imminent, health care had become a symbol of Canadian identity, and as such, a politically charged policy field. The political potency of health care has proven to be a serious constraint to change at a time when decision-making for health care requires dynamism and flexibility, rather than stability and stasis.

This approach to allocating health care ('rationing,' although the term is not popular in Canada's political vernacular) entails challenging, questioning, and altering the existing distributive paradigm. However, this is not equivalent to its rejection. The simple binary choices between universality and contingency, and solidarity and diversity seem to be inappropriate in the current context of health care reform. Contingent views of entitlement and respect for diversity can be reconciled with universality and solidarity. As will be explained in the next chapter, Marshall, the scholar credited with developing the notion of social rights, would encourage such revision and re-examination of citizenship arrangements.

2

Health Care Entitlement and Citizenship Development

Health is moving rapidly from the field of thinking of a service or a charity for some to be given by the better privileged to others ... into the field of thinking of it as an integral part of the life of every Canadian. In other words, the people are thinking of health as a right of citizenship, of even greater importance than education or police protection, which are taken for granted.

Canadian Federation of Agriculture, 1942[1]

I made a pledge with myself long before I ever sat in this House, in the years when I knew something about what it meant to get health services when you didn't have the money to pay for it. I made a pledge with myself that someday if I ever had anything to do with it, people would be able to get health services just as they are able to get educational services, as an inalienable right of being a citizen of a Christian country.

Tommy Douglas, 1962[2]

The support shown by Canadians for a universal, one-tier, single-payer health care system depends on their belief that it will provide to everyone, regardless of income, access to health care of the highest possible quality when that care is needed ... The perception and the reality of decline – and the worry about further decline to come presents us with one of the greatest public policy challenges facing this country today. After all, for Canadians, health care is not simply another government program. It has become tantamount to a right of citizenship. It reflects and it embodies some of the most fundamental values and principles of being a Canadian.

Federal Minister of Health, Allan Rock, 1997[3]

The above statements clearly indicate that health care in Canada is considered to be a right of citizenship. Patterns of entitlement were gradually institutionalized in the 1940s, 1950s, and 1960s, and now seem to be threatened by fiscal restraint measures, the neo-liberal trade agenda, and various reform efforts that have resulted in marginal erosion of the health system. In the face of such challenges, the right to health care is consistently defended. The bulwark that is created against retrenchment has a clear political message: citizens are entitled to universal health care, and they expect that their social rights will be protected regardless of changing economic circumstances. This might indeed be a reasonable and legitimate expectation. However, the political implications of repeated defences of the social rights thesis have been consistently neglected and need to be evaluated.[4]

Retrenching Health Care

In the 1980s and 1990s, governments in most advanced industrialized democracies were firmly committed to exercising fiscal restraint, which often meant retrenchment in the field of health care. Expenditures and demand for health care in Canada have grown steadily since the creation of national hospital and medical insurance programs in 1957 and 1966, respectively, and now seriously outpace governments' ability to provide adequate funding. As programs expanded throughout the post–Second World War decades, citizens' expectations rose continuously. People came to demand, as a matter of citizenship, virtually unlimited access to a comprehensive range of health services: this was partially the result of governments eagerly offering and delivering additional services within the popular universal health care system to secure voter support. By the mid-1970s this cycle of rising expectations and entitlement began to break down as governments came under pressure to contain costs in all areas. By 1977 the federal government replaced its generous intergovernmental cost-sharing arrangement with a block transfer, which allowed the federal government more control over its own spending in the field of health. In 1984 the Canada Health Act secured the federal government's role as defender of Canada's 'sacred trust.' Health care came to be an important symbol of national identity, which could now authoritatively be enforced (the act established the conditions on which transfer payments would continue to be disbursed to the provinces and the penalties for non-compliance).

From 1977 to the present, the federal government has reduced transfers to the provinces at the same time that it has continued to insist on compliance with (at least some of) the conditions specified in the Canada Health Act. Not surprisingly, this led to provincial resentment and subsequent demands for decentralization. Whether the federal government can, or should, maintain its role as defender of universal health care in Canada, and thereby strengthen the cohesive effects of health care as social right, or resign from its role and pass full decision-making authority to the provincial level and beyond is perhaps the most pressing political question of the day.[5] It is certainly of great importance to citizens who fear that the public system is in peril and that further retrenchment and federal abatement will make privatization (U.S. style) inevitable.

However, it is difficult to find solutions to Canada's health care crisis of funding, authority, and entitlement in the context of this ongoing debate. There is increasing ambiguity regarding levels of public support for universal health care. Federal and provincial governments engage in relentless and highly ideological wrangling to preserve Canada's sacred trust at the same time that they reduce spending commitments for health care. Politicians continuously misrepresent the principles, intentions, and limitations of the health care system and tend to cast debate in terms of impossible dichotomous choices. Such misrepresentation becomes legitimate as citizens resist changes to what they perceive to be their social rights of citizenship. Citizens consider a universally accessible, comprehensive set of portable benefits to be their right, and any attempts by politicians or bureaucrats to make changes in the system are considered a violation of rights. But how did this right develop? How is it changing? And is it still relevant at the beginning of the twenty-first century?

The symbolic appeal of health care and its importance as a feature of Canadian identity seem to have become institutionalized to such a degree that they constrain governmental decision-making. In the context of budgetary restraint, demographic changes, and technological advancement, such constraint is problematic. The defence of health care as a social right of citizenship is no longer a sufficient response to pressures for change.

It is entirely possible that the social rights thesis, propounded by T.H. Marshall in 1949, is no longer even relevant. Canada might be on the much feared and maligned slippery slope to health care business.

Health Canada reports that private expenditures now represent 30.1 per cent of all health expenditures,[6] and newspapers report that Canadian doctors are leaving the country to practise in the United States. In recent years, the Canadian Medical Association (CMA) has come close to formally supporting a two-tiered system, and there is a large faction within the medical profession that argues the position with conviction and authority on a regular basis. Marshall's inspiration, that citizenship is an evolving concept, has long been forgotten by defenders of the welfare state, and now serves only as a warning that should have been heeded, as approaches to health care provision in North America seem to be converging.

Health Politics in North American Perspective

The health system in the United States is considered to be one of the most inequitable and expensive in the industrialized world. Administrative costs, in addition to technological and demographic changes, have contributed to the rapid escalation of health care expenditures that now represent approximately 13.7 per cent of the U.S. gross domestic product (GDP).[7] Yet despite the rising costs and apparent expansion of the system, it is estimated that the percentage of uninsured workers age 19 to 64 who are not covered as a dependent or by a public program is approximately 23.3, and will increase to approximately 27 in 2005.[8] Governments, medical societies, employers, and citizens are well aware of the serious problems presented by an (arguably) well-funded health system that leaves a significant and growing proportion of the U.S. population uninsured, although there is no consensus on how the system should be reformed.

For Canadians, the universal health care system is a source of national pride, and an important symbol that distinguishes Canada from the United States.[9] Canadian health care reformers must exercise rhetorical caution in order that their efforts are not labelled 'Americanizations,' and Canadians seem to be relatively satisfied with their withering health care system because it is at least better than what is offered in the United States. Hence, the suggestion that a competitive market approach to health care would be feasible in Canada is counterintuitive, if not somewhat disturbing.

The pressure to adopt more market-type mechanisms in Canada has been staunchly and successfully resisted by Canadian reformers, and the social rights thesis has been consistently defended. However, the structure of the debate needs to be changed so that it is no longer an ideological one between those on the social democratic left who defend social rights as a remedy to inequality, and those on the right who argue that social rights are an affront to responsibility, efficiency, and freedom of choice. The social rights thesis needs to be more thoroughly critiqued and revised from the left, rather than merely defended with various caveats. The social rights thesis is outmoded. It has been critiqued and revised rigorously only from the right by those seeking to limit entitlements for 'undeserving' citizens.

Lawrence Mead, for example, argues that 'a policy of enforcing work and other civilities [in the United States] is the truest to Marshall's idea, and also the most effective.'[10] In other words, Marshall's understanding of citizenship includes a citizen–state exchange of entitlements and duties. At this point, Mead's argument is exactly right. As I will explain later in this chapter, and throughout the rest of the book, Marshall did intend that social rights would be tied to duties. In fact, Marshall may even have thought duties of citizenship to be primary. It was because citizens served the state through the military or the workforce that some type of compensation was their due. This compensation would be guaranteed as a matter of citizenship, and not contingent on social class, charity, or the benevolence of welfare case workers.

According to Mead, those who follow Marshall tend to 'emphasize the claims of citizenship,' and ignore the importance of obligations.[11] This creates a problem in that the recipients of social entitlements are simply assumed to be 'deserving.'[12] Mead explains that 'what legitimizes social insurance programs is their strong tie to employment. The beneficiaries of unemployment, pension, and health benefits, or their employers, pay premiums while they are working. They then may claim support from the programs with few questions asked when, due to layoff, age, or infirmity, they cannot work.'[13]

Mead's analysis is consistent with what I will call Marshall's weaker vision. Marshall argues that the state should provide 'a modicum of economic welfare and security.'[14] This might include such 'safety net' programs as welfare assistance, disability insurance, wage subsidies, and unemployment benefits. In constructing his case against the continued generous disbursement of welfare payments to malingering claimants, Mead employs Marshall's weaker vision for support. By linking the citizen duties that Marshall identifies to the weaker vision of state obligation, Mead is able to demonstrate that unless a particular citizen works, she or he is not eligible, according to Marshall's criteria, to receive the safety net benefits (such as unemployment assistance). This is an absurd argument, and one that indicates a serious misinterpretation of Marshall's social rights thesis.

First, if a particular citizen is working, then it is unlikely that she or he will require unemployment benefits or welfare payments. Second, Mead's reasoning fails to take into account Marshall's stronger vision. The complete idea of social rights is that the state will recognize 'the whole range from the right to a modicum of economic welfare and security to the right to share to the full in the social heritage and to live the life of a civilized being according to the standards prevailing in the society.'[15]

The degree to which social rights have been institutionalized in the United States is limited. With the main exceptions of Social Security (pension benefits) and Medicare parts A and B (hospital and medical insurance for seniors), there are no social programs to which all citizens are entitled on equal terms and conditions. Furthermore, it is quite clear that in this stronger vision, Marshall is concerned with societies and the citizenship arrangements that define them, not with the compliance or deviance of particular individuals. Mead seems to be obsessed with determining what to do with individuals who 'choose' a freeloading life of non-work over fulfilling their duties of citizenship. This might indeed be a problem that requires thorough investigation. But it is not, in my view, a question that can be addressed by Marshall.

Those on the left need to recognize that new challenges, such as those posed by differentiated citizenship, are not satisfied by the simple promise of equality that is inherent in social rights. The changing nature of after claims and constitutional and citizenship arrangements alter the context and substance of social rights. In addition, health care as a community and social right, institutionalized in conditions of relaxed scarcity and political commitments to Keynesianism, is running headlong into legal rights claims and the vagaries of budgeting in periods of chronic and acute scarcity.[16]

Moreover, the right to health care has become institutionalized as a potent political symbol in Canada. The political importance of health care makes governments reluctant to significantly alter patterns of service provision, even when there is evidence to indicate that change is necessary (i.e. it might be necessary to eliminate overlapping and inefficient services, but hospital closures result in public outcry). That the social rights thesis is outmoded does not mean that the market approach to health care is either inevitable or fair; Marshall's essay needs to be updated to clarify and strengthen commitments to equality, not overturn them. The institutionalization and continued uncritical defence of social rights in Canada has caused stasis, and presents a stumbling block to discursive and policy progress.

Revisiting the Social Rights Thesis

Social rights developed as the result of the confluence of many social, political, and economic factors. It is not surprising that citizens came to consider universal health care to be their right; health care was established as an entitlement program (as opposed to means tested, for example). Enrolment in the public plan was guaranteed as a matter of citizenship, and citizens considered these social benefits to be 'their due': recognition and compensation by the state for the difficult times endured throughout the 1930s and 1940s. Furthermore, and again in the language of rights, citizens 'justly expected'[17] that the recent advances in medical technology would be made available to all, on an equal basis. The 'bargain' that was struck between citizens and the state, which entailed relatively high rates of taxation and heavy regulation of the economy in return for social programs, was maintained for approximately three decades (1945–77). As the politico-economic climate changed throughout the postwar decades, it became apparent that citizens' expectations do not easily adjust downward, especially when the burdens of citizenship (taxes, restraint, unemployment) are high. Health care has become an important social program (because it distributes much-needed services and mitigates inequality of status) as well as a powerful political symbol.

However, the promise of social rights, namely, the guarantee of a minimum standard of citizenship to secure substantive equality, is somewhat empty. Contemporary citizenship is marked by increasing differentiation and requires variable definitions of political equality. According to identity theorists, welfare state political commitments to equality and universality have been only marginally successful in delivering substantive citizenship benefits.[18] For while equal procedural rights have been accorded to all citizens, gains in equal substance of citizenship have been thin. The rhetorical force of the former tends to diminish the claims concerning the latter. An empty promise that continues to constrain much-needed reform efforts should raise concern. It should also present a paradox in that health care, as Canada's most important social program, might be undermined by its strength as a political symbol.

The need to revise the social rights thesis is not so much a critique of its original formulator, Marshall, as it is a critique of those who have interpreted and advanced the idea of social rights as citizenship. In his 1949 essay, 'Citizenship and Social Class,' Marshall examines the compatibility of formal rights of citizenship with social class, and argues that 'the inequality of the social class system may be acceptable provided the equality of citizenship is recognized.'[19] In the twentieth century, equality of citizenship was guaranteed through the provision of social services.

To fully understand how Marshall explains the historical evolution of citizenship, it is necessary to revisit his analysis and retrace the lines that link social class to rights possession. The relationship between social class and rights has not always been grounded in assumptions of political equality. The notion that all human beings are entitled to certain inalienable rights (and ought to be entitled to a range of social rights) is only a few hundred years old, and it has not been formally endorsed in all democratic nations.

The general theme of Marshall's argument, hereafter referred to as the social rights thesis, is well known. Marshall explains that there are three 'elements' of citizenship, that have been 'dictated by history even more clearly than by logic.'[20] These are the civil, political, and social:

> The civil element is composed of the rights necessary for individual freedom – liberty of the person, freedom of speech, thought, and faith, the right to own property and to conclude valid contracts, and the right to justice ... By the political element I mean the right to participate in the exercise of political power, as a member of a body invested with political authority or as an elector of the members of such a body ... By the social element I mean the whole range from the right to a modicum of economic welfare and security to the right to share to the full in the social heritage and to live the life of a civilized being according to the standards prevailing in the society.[21]

According to Marshall, these elements of citizenship did not develop in mutual exclusion, although it is possible to identify their moments of congealment in the eighteenth, nineteenth, and twentieth centuries, respectively. Each element of citizenship, or type of right, is aimed at minimizing inequality in social status so that every citizen will be able to fulfil his or her duties, and thereby be accorded full membership in the political community.

That social rights could guarantee equal status of citizenship regardless of social class (wealth or income level) was a grand promise. Indeed, Marshall's historical and normative analysis of the development of citizenship provides theoretical foundations for countless arguments both in defence and repudiation of the welfare state. However, the complexities of Marshall's argument are either outmoded or seriously underdeveloped by those who have popularized the social rights thesis.

On the first charge, that the social rights thesis is outmoded, there are two main points to be made. Marshall is concerned about limiting the effects of class distinctions. He believes that all citizens should have equal status, regardless of social class: 'social rights imply an absolute right to a certain standard of civilization which is conditional only on the discharge of the general duties of citizenship. Their content does not depend on the economic value of the individual claimant.'[22] So, first, it is important to notice that Marshall considers social class to be the primary source of inequality among citizens. Certainly, class abatement was an important achievement, on which many other social gains (in the direction of equality) were contingent. However, 50 years after Marshall's lectures, it is not at all clear whether social rights, as both a theoretical construct and a pragmatic political promise, can accommodate or mitigate more profound and immeasurable forms of inequality (such as those based on gender, sexual orientation, race, and ability). Jytte Klausen has argued that 'it is erroneous to regard social citizenship as the equivalent of civil and political rights and that instead it is necessary to distinguish between rights and redistribution. Social rights imply redistribution of income between social groups ... [and as such, social rights have proved to be] a suggestive metaphor for political mobilization aimed at putting together broadly based coalitions on behalf of welfare state expansion.'[23] Although the notion of redistributive compensation for socially disadvantaged groups is bound up in the meaning of social rights, social rights are, indeed, rights.

Second, in Canada, the promise that equality could be delivered through social programs, namely, universal health care, became institutionalized as a highly charged political symbol. That all Canadian citizens should have access to a comprehensive range of health care services seems to be a non-negotiable, self-evident tenet of the state–

society relationship. Hence, government efforts to restructure the health care system are often construed as an affront to the social rights of citizenship.

Careful political posturing is necessary so that changes can be made without causing alarm among the electorate. On the one hand, the institutionalization of social rights has a positive effect, in that the benefits conferred by social rights (to achieve equal status of citizenship), universal health insurance being the most prized, cannot easily be rescinded by governments. On the other hand, however, the political importance of universal health care constrains governments in constructing a viable reform agenda. It is this negative effect that indicates the need to revise, rather than continue to blindly defend, the social rights thesis. Such a suggestion does not render Marshall's analysis useless. Rather, it makes necessary clarification of Marshall's original argument, separation of it from those of his defenders, and careful revision.

The second charge, that defenders of the social rights thesis have either misinterpreted Marshall's argument, or failed to revise it, is confined here to analysis of the health care system in Canada, although it also has global implications. Those scholars and practitioners concerned about the erosion of the welfare state by the forces of globalization, catalyzed by a neo-liberal trade agenda (environmentalists, nationalists, those who defend borders as a means of protecting hard-won social policies, for example), have little choice but to come to terms with what they perceive to be threatening forces, and find new ways to defend or promote their interests within that context. Similarly, those scholars who categorically defend the social rights thesis misunderstand the dynamics of change that have to be considered within the definition of citizenship, and need to recast their arguments in accordance with fiscal, administrative, demographic, and ethical pressures for reform. Prolonged, uncritical defence can do real damage, because it serves to reinforce the strength of health care as a political symbol regardless of the imperatives for change.

The main problem is that defenders fail to recognize that social rights might unduly protect existing patterns of authority and provision of services (namely, the dominance of the medical profession and the preference for institutional care). Social rights hold constant the mechanics and structure of the health care system. This might be further simplified to say that between periods of comprehensive policy change, there is a degree of 'path dependency' that accounts for stability in policy development.[24] Such stability in the Canadian context is both beneficial and burdensome, the ambivalence conveniently bound up in health care rights claims.

Canadian scholars and casual observers seem to have too much faith in the ability of social rights to equalize the status of citizenship, and such faith is becoming less and less feasible as the contours of citizenship, economics, and health care change. Continued rights claims in regard to health care are problematic for both the theoretical and political inconsistencies that they present. Conceptually, current patterns of health care rights claims are disjunctive with what Marshall envisioned, in that they are increasingly individualistic, and Marshall's thesis has not been revised to sufficiently recognize identity rights. Politically, social rights, as the embodiment of citizens' expectations for continued development of welfare state programs, hold little promise in contemporary intergovernmental, budgetary, medical, and epidemiological contexts.

Defending the Social Rights Thesis: Problems and Puzzles

There are two main problems with the social rights thesis: It is dated, and has become institutionalized in Canada to such an extent that it causes stasis. In addition, there are a number of specific reasons why the social rights thesis is outmoded, and hence problematic as an entrenched component of Canadian citizenship.

1 Marshall's historical narrative and conceptual argument pertain directly to Britain. Over the past 50 years, the social rights thesis has become, seemingly, universally applicable, yet it has not been well developed to fit with, or describe, circumstances in other countries or temporal periods.
2 Similarly, Marshall might have originally intended his analysis to have equal relevance for all components of the 'right to a modicum of economic welfare and security to the right to share to the full in the social heritage and to live ... life ... according to the standards prevailing in the society,' but most contemporary discussions of social rights address issues of poverty or education. Thus, to evaluate the right to health care as a sub-entitlement of social rights, further modifications and specifications must be made.
3 Marshall's one-dimensional understanding of inequality, as the result of social class differences, does not fully account for inequality

in multi-ethnic, multicultural states. Various critiques and discussions further probe this problem, but, even taken together, they are not sufficiently specific (to country or policy field) and do not address the political implications of new sources of inequality or the perpetuation of old ones.

For example, J.M. Barbalet considers the intersection of class inequality and rights struggle.[25] Barbalet submits that Marshall's contribution to citizenship discourse is unparalleled, nevertheless, imperfect for a number of reasons, the most important of which is that Marshall underestimates the divisive effects of social class. Specifically, the social rights thesis fails to recognize the degree to which inequalities in wealth and income create barriers to the exercise of rights. Marshall is unconcerned with the logic of capitalism, and he addresses only the effects of markets as a means of achieving substantive political equality. Barbalet argues that this is merely glossing over class inequality and may, as such, exacerbate rather than mitigate that inequality.

The problem under discussion remains class inequality, which might currently have greater relevance in Britain than in Canada. Class is one of many cleavages in Canada, but not, arguably, the most politically divisive or salient. Language, region, gender, and sexual orientation intersect with class, and the elimination or reduction of inequalities generated by these differences is contingent in many cases on class abatement. Consideration of social class, then, as the sole determinant of inequality is problematic in twenty-first century North America.

This problem is addressed by Bryan Turner and Barry Hindness,[26] who demonstrate a sound understanding of the social rights thesis, yet recognize the importance of incorporating a differentiated perspective in discussions of social citizenship. Hindness's critique from the left is particularly compelling. He argues that equality has not been achieved by the institutionalization of social rights, and gains that have been made through political commitments to social rights and under the rubric of equal status of citizenship do not sufficiently close the gap between citizenship and social class, and reinforce certain traditional familial patterns. Neither Hindness nor Turner consider the political implications of either model of citizenship.

4 The development of social rights in the postwar period was, in part, the result of the macroeconomic trends of that time. Commitments to

Keynesianism, as part of the Bretton Woods Agreement, allowed governments to spend on social programs regardless of budgetary circumstances. The feasibility of such an approach declined in the 1970s, and by the 1990s, balancing the budget had become the priority of virtually all Canadian governments. The macroeconomic trends of the period in which social rights were developed are markedly different from those of the period in which social rights – as health care rights claims – are being defended. This deserves examination. Most contemporary discussions have neglected to do so.

5 The need for social rights, specifically, universal health care, was pressing in the period of social rights development because of the prevailing dynamics of health and disease. State action was necessary in the 1940s and 1950s as a response to public health epidemics and the prevalence of communicable diseases. In the current context, the main causes of death and serious illness are non-communicable diseases. This change has profound social effects. This shift in the main causes of death, from communicable to non-communicable diseases, in addition to trends of deinstitutionalization – which leave home care and pharmaceuticals (sometimes prohibitively expensive) – outside 'universal' programs, requires a new blend of individual responsibility and collective entitlement, as well as more differentiated approaches to the delivery of services.

6 Marshall conceived of social citizenship as a reciprocal arrangement between citizens and the state. The implications of such reciprocity have not been thoroughly examined or sufficiently understood in contemporary defences of the social rights thesis. Desmond King and Jeremy Waldron, for example, recognize that there is tight reciprocity between social rights and duties, but they do not evaluate this correlation.[27] At the heart of their analysis is the assumption that social rights constitute legitimate expectations. This assumption, concerning the normative claim that citizens are entitled to social benefits, is valid, but the implications of the claim need further examination. King and Waldron's uncritical assessment serves to maintain the polarization of statist and market approaches to addressing social inequality. Their argument, structured as a debate between proponents of social rights theory and the New Right, gives the impression that social rights can either be defended, or rejected outright: no middle ground is available in their argument, just a tug-of-war between ideologues.

Marshall's description of the development of social rights and his suggestion that states ought to institutionalize social rights as a matter of citizenship, are contingent on his historical analysis, which finds that rights were accorded by governments in a piecemeal way, and in response to the requirements of capitalism.

This is an important point, and one that has been almost completely ignored by Marshall's followers. In the eighteenth century, the basic civil right in the economic field was the right to work,

> that is to say the right to follow the occupation of one's choice, subject only to legitimate demands for preliminary technical training. This right had been denied by both statute and custom; on the one hand by the Elizabethan Statute of Artificers, which confined certain occupations to certain social classes, and on the other by local regulations reserving employment in a town to its own members and by the use of apprenticeship as an instrument of exclusion rather than recruitment. The recognition of the right involved the formal acceptance of a fundamental change of attitude. The old assumption that local and group monopolies were in the public interest, because 'trade and traffic cannot be maintained or increased without order and government,' was replaced by the new assumption that such restrictions were an offence against the liberty of the subject and a menace to the prosperity of the nation.[28]

The right to work (as an expression of liberty), and the duty to exercise that right, were secured (through the courts) because they were essential to the economic well-being of the nation. In the next century, political rights were also won (by certain segments of the population) through economic struggle; the right to vote, or stand for political office, were necessary for citizens to protect their private property, and participate in decision-making that would affect their right to work. And it was because economic liberalism required an educated and healthy populace that the rights to education and health care were granted to all British citizens, regardless of social class, in the twentieth century.

With the institutionalization of the first part of Marshall's citizenship equation (rights), a certain passive conception of equality was engendered. The duty side of the equation creates a more active conception of equality, which has become appealing to both left- and right-wing proponents of change. Health reform agendas in the Canadian provinces harbour these competing notions of equality, which makes difficult the implementation of coherent reform measures.

Social Rights and the Politics of Difference

Here, it is necessary to briefly explain how the debate concerning the politics of difference is relevant to discussions of health care, entitlement, and the role of the state. Identity theorists, such as Iris Marion Young, do not question the principles of democracy or pluralism, but are critical of the ways in which they are operationalized.[29] The promise of equality of citizens in influencing political decisions is theoretically sound, yet practically problematic. Procedural guarantees need to be combined with recognition, through public policy, of substantive differences among citizens and groups of citizens. The mechanisms through which recognition could be institutionalized might, for instance, include 'public funds for advocacy groups, guaranteed representation in political bodies, and veto rights over specific policies that affect a group directly.'[30] Such an approach could help to address historical patterns of marginalization, as well as allow for a more effective distribution of resources.

This approach is mainly a challenge from contemporary and feminist political theory to incorporate identity and difference into dominant cultural and political systems. Differentiated citizenship claims, or identity rights, enrich the conceptual debate over social rights and citizenship, and offer a thoroughgoing critique of welfare state patterns of entitlement. They also provide a model for rethinking health care policy in a context of insufficient resources (i.e., government funding) and rising citizen expectations. Different communities (the elderly, women, persons with HIV/AIDS) need to use the health care system in varying ways, and public policy should reflect these differences, not dissolve them into existing programs. This does not suggest repudiating universality, but building on it in new ways. There already are different services and programs available for Native Canadians, people with diseases that require prohibitively expensive medications, and the elderly (who have drug entitlements that are not available to the general Canadian population). This approach needs to be expanded, and such an expansion might pull the health care system out of its current 'static' position.

What I am suggesting also requires a complete rethinking of the Canadian social citizenship bargain. It is possible to continue to distribute health care as a public good in Canada, but a fair distribution no longer denotes a strictly equal distribution. 'Political communities,' as the basis for understanding the population's health care needs and delivering on them, need to be reconceived as identity-based so that they can inform and interact with geographically based decision-making entities. This strategy will be discussed more thoroughly in Chapter 7.

Conclusion

The social rights thesis, as conceptualized in this chapter, provides the standard welfare state entitlement approach against which public policy issues and problems are evaluated. In Chapters 3 and 4, the meaning and implications of the right to health care in Canada will be explained and addressed so that in the successive institutional- and policy-oriented chapters it can be determined to what extent the institutionalization of universal entitlement has proven to be a barrier to system reform and policy progress.

3

The Evolution of Social Rights in Canada

The resonance of T.H. Marshall's work on citizenship is remarkable. In a series of lectures, Marshall was able to cogently explain the evolution of citizenship over three centuries, and, at the same time, capture the essence of contemporary and emerging sentiment concerning social inequality and entitlement. However, the social rights thesis has been consistently defended as an infungible, sustainable element of the state–society relationship, in spite of Marshall's caveat that citizenship is an evolving concept. In this chapter I examine closely Marshall's third stage of citizenship development – social rights – to evaluate the extent of change in Canadian social and political contexts and the consequent transformation of the right to health care.

Such an exercise will serve to address three main problems with contemporary defences of the social rights thesis. First, Marshall's analysis, intended specifically as a historical analysis and set of normative claims pertaining directly to Great Britain in the immediate post–Second World War period, has been imported to other geographic and temporal contexts without careful consideration of how the meaning and substance of citizenship rights developed in different countries over time. Second, although Marshall mentions health care as one component of the citizenship bargain, his historical narrative clearly deals with issues of poverty and the need for inclusive measures of poor relief. Therefore, to make a case about the right to health care, further modifications to the social rights thesis must be made. These modifications would include, among others, evaluation of different policy areas (namely, health care), countries (in historical context), political systems (federal), cultural dynamics, and temporal periods. And third, in the Canadian context it is likely that citizenship is developing beyond the social rights period. The simple unity that was generated by the implementation of universal social programs has become dissonant with emerging, differentiated citizenship claims.

To examine these problems, I will offer answers to the following questions: How did the right to health care become institutionalized in Canada, and how has it evolved since the immediate postwar period? In this chapter, I will argue that the meaning of the right to health care (as a subset of social rights) has changed significantly in Canada throughout the past 50 or 60 years, and currently embodies competing individual and collective dimensions.

Social Rights as Citizenship

There are generally considered to be two periods of social rights development in Canada. The first is a 'relatively stable citizenship regime that lasted from the 1940s to the 1980s.'[1] In this period the 'federal government funded a wide range of citizen groups that were seen as the vehicles for helping disadvantaged segments of the population achieve equality through collective action and, in so doing, reaffirm their Canadian identity.'[2] Also, in this period many important social programs were created and 'were generally pan-Canadian in nature, supported by the use of the federal spending power.'[3] These programs drastically altered the citizenship regime; what it meant to be Canadian evolved in this period to include access to a range of social benefits. The universal health care system would become the most revered of the social programs.

The commencement of the second period is marked by promulgation of the Canadian Charter of Rights and Freedoms in 1982. Katherine Graham and Susan Phillips explain that 'on the one hand, the Charter made a commitment to "categorical equity." Women, the disabled, aboriginal peoples were designated as categories of citizens who should receive *equitable* treatment. On the other hand, the Charter entrenched individual rights and provided a reference point for the emerging philosophy of individual responsibility taking.'[4]

The latter points to an individualistic turn in Canadian rights culture. Regarding health care, this has contributed greatly to the shift in citizens' expectations that is discernible today. As governments continue to exercise fiscal restraint, levels of service are declining. The implication of this harsh reality, in addition to the emergence of a more individualistic rights culture, is that disjunction is created in the distribution of the benefits and burdens of citizenship. Moreover, as social rights are diminished in the context of retrenchment, citizens are making legalistic and possessive individualistic rights claims in the hope of preserving the social rights regime. This is itself a paradox because social rights are rooted in a normative/objective conception of right, and modern, possessive conceptions are a major departure from this. These philosophical distinctions are addressed in Chapter 4.

The Charter's commitment to 'categorical equity' also demands consideration in this debate. While rights have become more individualistic, the legal recognition of social inequality based on gender, race, and sexual orientation, has created new definitions of 'community' and identified more sources of inequality – other than social class. Thus, the requirements of citizenship in Canada and other Western democracies are becoming greater in number and diversity, which make it less likely that the promise of simple unity through universal access to social goods as a matter of citizenship obtains in current and future social, political, and economic contexts. This is not to say that universal health care provision is no longer important. It is. The point here is that the social rights thesis needs to be revised so that it can provide an appropriate theoretical context for reform, rather than an obstacle to debate and action.

Health Care: Canada's Collective Conscience

Perhaps the most important information about the first period of social rights development is economic. This was a period of 'relaxed scarcity';[5] there was nearly full employment, and the postwar economy was strong. Government had acquired the means necessary to mitigate the effects of the Great Depression, which proved that everyone was vulnerable to economic adversity, regardless of social class. The 44 per cent rejection rate of young male recruits for the war effort further demonstrated the need for national action in health care because those in poor health could not fulfil their military obligation to their country.[6]

The development of the universal health care system began with the report of the Rowell-Sirois Commission on Dominion-Provincial Relations, which recommended state medical insurance.[7] This recommendation was a reflection of the growing need for health care services among the populace, as well as the recognition, in the aftermath of the Great Depression, that provincial governments might not have the revenue capacity sufficient to fund social initiatives. Furthermore, it was the view of the commission that 'the necessary solvent, the circumstance under which enough consensus results to make federalism workable, is thus widely distributed economic well-being.'[8] In other words, redistribution was important not only as a matter of fairness, but because it was required by the federal state.

The commission was also prudent to recognize that federal involvement in areas of provincial jurisdiction was a volatile undertaking. In 1937, the same year that the Rowell-Sirois Commission was appointed, the Judicial Committee of the Privy Council (JCPC) declared most of former Prime Minister R.B. Bennett's New Deal legislation to be *ultra vires*. The purpose of the New Deal was to provide relief to Canadians who had suffered through the depression, as well as to create a social vision for the country. Even though Bennett's legislation was not passed, it marked the beginning of a new era of social policy in Canada.

Then, in 1947, the Co-operative Commonwealth Federation (CCF) government in Saskatchewan became the first provincial government to institute a public hospital insurance program. This was a particularly bold move since the federal government had not yet committed itself to the establishment of a national hospital insurance program or to support provincial initiatives. The CCF government, led by Premier Tommy Douglas, had campaigned on the promise to implement a hospital insurance plan, and fulfilled the promise two and one half years into its mandate, in spite of deadlocked federal–provincial relations on the issue. The pioneer legislation was the product of the culmination of many economic factors as well as new political forces. Municipal doctor and hospital plans were failing because of the inadequacy of provincial resources; the citizens of Saskatchewan were desperate for a competent public health care system. Clearly, Saskatchewan farmers' duty to work was contingent on their own health, and that of their families. Harley Dickinson explains:

> Agricultural production in Canada in general, and Saskatchewan in particular, is based on production for the market. It is not primarily organized on a subsistence basis. Consequently farmers' incomes depend upon farmer productivity on the one hand, and relative market strength on the other. Anything that threatens productive capacity, including injury or illness, also threatens the economic well-being and survival of farmers. Because Saskatchewan farmers are both owners of capital in the

form of land and equipment, and dependent on the use of their own and family members unpaid labour to produce crops, they have a direct interest in ensuring the quality and productive capacity of that labour power. Medical and hospital services, in addition to other illness and injury prevention programs and health care services, are important in this regard.[9]

The CCF party's commitment to public health insurance recognized these issues and in so doing generated subsequent demand among other sectors of the population. In 1962 political conviction and broad public support led to the development of public medical services insurance in Saskatchewan; again, this was the first such program in Canada.

In 1957 the Canadian federal government implemented a national hospital insurance program. The federal contribution for hospital insurance was allocated to the provinces on a cost-matching basis; 25 per cent of the cost of national average per capita hospital services and 25 per cent average per capita costs in the particular province, multiplied by the number of insured persons.[10] The conditions of the program were perceived by the provincial governments as a massive intrusion into a field of exclusive provincial jurisdiction, although the program itself was heralded as a victory for the provinces.[11]

In any case, the federal government, following Saskatchewan's lead, had begun the process by which universal hospital and medical insurance would be institutionalized as components of Canadian citizenship.

The health care system was being transformed from a parochial arrangement of citizens, communities, churches, doctors, and other caregivers, with informal obligations to one another, to a state-managed program of universally accessible health services, to which all citizens were formally entitled. During the period of informal obligations, the right to health care translated as the expectation that communicable diseases and other public health issues would be brought under control, and that a range of advanced medical services would be available in Canada for private consumption. In the period of public health care insurance, the right to health care indicated the expectation that hospital and medical services would be distributed as public goods. Health care as social right was essential for the prosperity of the country, the levelling of social class differences (perhaps the most significant cleavage of the time), and, eventually, the formation of national identity.

In 1943 the Canadian Medical Association (CMA) endorsed, in principle, a national health insurance program, and seemed to be quite willing to comply with governments' formalization and institutionalization of the right to health care. The historical record shows that, in 1943, 'during the public hearings of the [House of Commons Select] Committee on Social Security, the CMA gave a ringing endorsement of the proposed national program, assuring the Committee that the profession would "render any assistance in its power towards the solution of one of the country's most important problems."'[12] However, because of political inaction on the issue, physicians organized themselves to develop prepayment schemes, thereby pre-empting the public health insurance programs that would come into effect in the next two decades.

The 1945 Green Book Proposals of the federal government, which had outlined an intergovernmental approach to health care in which the federal government would take a lead role, effectively 'foundered in the failure of the Dominion–Provincial Conference on Post War Reconstruction 1945–46, at which federal-provincial agreement could not be reached on the transfer of tax fields to the federal government to finance the measures.'[13]

The willingness of the medical profession to take action to address the problems of inadequate access to health services and difficulty securing adequate remuneration for physicians, in addition to the intergovernmental inertia in the immediate postwar period, 'enabled the profession to make giant leaps in establishing profession-controlled prepayment plans to fill the vacuum.'[14]

The prepayment plans, established and administered by professional associations in conjunction with the commercial insurance industry, insured patients against sickness and injury, which effectively improved access; citizens now had choice in planning financially for their health care (an issue of grave importance in the aftermath of the depression). They also guaranteed some remuneration for physicians who were adversely affected by economic uncertainty.

As a result of continued government inaction and the rapid expansion of the prepayment plans, by 1949 the CMA had reversed its decision to endorse national (public) health insurance. Malcolm Taylor explains: 'While continuing to support the objective of health insurance it now declared that the role of government should be limited simply to paying to the voluntary plans the premiums, in whole or in part, on behalf of those unable to pay the full amount.'[15] Clearly, the commercial benefit of these voluntary plans had shaped the interests of organized medicine in health care. The medical associations became quite comfortable with their newly acquired 'private government'[16] status, and were prepared to defend it against what they perceived to be encroachment by the state. By 1947 a public hospital insurance program had been successfully implemented in Saskatchewan, followed by similar action on a national level exactly one decade later. Malcolm Taylor, Michael Stevenson, and Paul Williams explain:

> The success of national hospital insurance by the end of the 1950s focussed public attention on the issue of medical care and the prepayment plans were, in a sense, the victims of their own success. They had proved that medical care insurance was as desirable and workable as hospital insurance but they, together with the commercial insurance industry, had been able to insure less than half the population (10.6 million in 1965).[17]

The medical associations that demonstrated competence in the health insurance field indicated to governments that public programs would be similarly viable. Moreover, the equity issue loomed large, as the voluntary prepayment plans did not cover the entire Canadian population. This issue was presented as a glaring injustice in the 1964 report of the Hall Commission, which directed the federal government to extend the benefits of available technology to the entire population as a matter of social right.

Great Expectations: The Royal Commission on Health Services

The Royal Commission on Health Services (Hall Commission, 1961–4)[18] is, perhaps, the most important milestone in the history of the Canadian health care system, for two reasons: (1) It was remarkably comprehensive and ahead of its time. The Hall Report presented a very advanced view of the future of the Canadian health care system: (2) Many of its recommendations were implemented.

The primary concern of the commission was that the benefits of new medical technology be extended to the entire Canadian population. Prior to 1957 there were a variety of health insurance plans in the provinces, which included both hospital and medical benefits. In 1957 the Hospital Insurance and Diagnostic Act implemented a broad, universal program that subsumed many of the existing grants-in-aid (which were established under the National Health Grants Program, 1948), such as the Hospital Construction Grant, and grants for tuberculosis control, mental health, venereal disease, children with disabilities, and cancer among others. Within the succeeding decade, communicable diseases such as venereal disease, tuberculosis, and smallpox were largely under control, and a more comprehensive health care program was needed. With new medical developments, all of these diseases (and many others) could be controlled, and, therefore, it was believed that they should be controlled as a matter of social or community right.

The success and popularity of the national hospital services program generated demand for a comprehensive public medical insurance plan. The Hall Commission reported: 'With almost the total population becoming entitled to prepaid hospital services, the next essential service to be organized is care provided by physicians and surgeons and some ancillary services all of which we refer to as "medical services."'[19] It was recommended that these services be provided by physicians on a fee-for-service basis, which was closer to the U.S. (private) model than the U.K. model, in which consultant physicians were salaried employees of the state and general practitioners were paid on a capitalization basis.

The commission's terms of reference focused on individual responsibility for health and well-being at the same time that they recognized the importance of the needs of the community. The areas that were designated to be matters of public interest were environmental controls (including clean drinking water, sewer systems, communicable disease control), education of health care professionals, health care facilities, personnel, and universal availability and access to services.[20] Regarding the public interest in individual health, the Commission stated: 'The public interest in individual health has been typically manifested by community action to deal with health problems that the individual was incapable of managing himself. In the past this meant community measures to prevent and control communicable diseases. Organized health activities in Canada originated in community efforts to stem the epidemics of the last century.'[21]

The contours of communicable disease required that collective action be taken. C.E.S. Franks explains that early government action in public health included commitments to 'sewerage systems, pest control, assurance of pure water supply, pasteurization of milk, meat and food inspection, sanitary inspection of public eating establishments, public conveyances and the like.'[22] These areas were considered to be within the realm of public responsibility because they could not be dealt with by individual citizens. It would have been unreasonable to expect water purification systems or sewers to be installed on an individual basis. Such measures are only advantageous if they are undertaken by every member of the community. Public health cannot be improved if some homes are supplied with water purification systems and sewers, and others not; if some milk is subject to the pasteurization process and some is not; if some meat is inspected and some is not; or if some people are immunized against communicable diseases and some are not. In this way, these public health services are properly regarded to be community rights, exercised by communities on behalf of their constituents.

In contrast to the differentiated group rights that will be discussed in a subsequent section (such rights define the fourth stage of citizenship development in Canada: identity rights), these examples are definitive of universal community rights. In the case of the latter, all citizens are equally entitled, and equally benefited, and individual responsibility-taking is an issue of secondary importance.

Universality Congealed: National Medical Insurance

The Health Charter for Canadians, proposed by the Hall Commission, brought into being the terms of the National Medical Insurance Plan. It states that the objectives of health policy 'can best be achieved through a comprehensive, universal Health Services Program for the Canadian people,' which will be implemented in accordance with 'Canada's evolving constitutional arrangements,' and recognizes the right to 'freedom of choice' to be exercised by individual patients and practitioners.[23] The problematic broadness and symbolic importance of these terms would become major and controversial issues soon after the implementation of the plan.

The arrangements for public medical insurance (1966) established that the federal government would pay 50 per cent 'of the national per capita cost of insured services, multiplied by the insured population of the province,'[24] and the provinces were required to operate programs in accordance with federally determined standards. However, there were many problems with the shared-cost funding arrangement. Paul Barker explains:

> The reasons for uncontrolled growth in costs were easy to detect. One was the open-endedness of the arrangements. The only limit was the ability of

the provinces to spend. Another was the matching element, which provided an incentive for provinces to spend on shared-cost programs. A
further reason was that the federal government often shared with the
provinces only the most expensive services.

Under this kind of arrangement, the provinces had little incentive to
develop more efficient ways of delivering services ... The federal government shared only in the cost of expensive hospital and medical care,
which in turn inhibited the development of less expensive but equally
effective health care.[25]

The development of 'less expensive but equally effective health care'
would become the goal of health care reformers in the 1990s. During
the formative years of the national health plan, however, other objectives, such as improving the health of Canadians, guaranteeing access
for all citizens regardless of socioeconomic status, and ensuring a fair
distribution of the benefits and burdens of citizenship in a technologi-
cally advanced democracy, were paramount.

In the first nine years of the program, the provinces held the balance
of power because they had the ability, by virtue of the financing
arrangements, to determine total (federal and provincial) spending on
health care services. However, the 1970s were marked by increased
need for the federal government to improve planning in all policy
areas as well as by the strengthening of provincial autonomy claims. In
this context, the implementation of Established Programs Financing
(EPF) to replace the cost-matching arrangements began to shift the
focus of the debate from accessibility criteria to efficiency and effectiveness criteria. This meant that the right to health care, initially guaranteed in rather open-ended terms, was being increasingly subject to
limits. Most obviously, entitlement was constrained by budgetary
planning and belt-tightening. At the same time, fiscal planning and
belt-tightening measures were constrained by the popularity, in both
practical and symbolic terms, of the universal health system.

Towards Scarcity and Stasis

Not surprisingly, with the increasingly volatile political situation of the
1970s came a change in federal–provincial fiscal arrangements. In 1977
the federal government implemented EPF which unilaterally altered
the intergovernmental funding arrangements for health care and post-
secondary education. The purpose of EPF was to discontinue the prac-

tice of provincial governments determining federal spending levels through shared-cost arrangements, thereby enabling the federal government's budgetary planning initiatives. In addition, it was a response to provincial demands for relaxed conditionality of federal funds. The federal government was able to make concessions to provincial governments (amid the volatility of province-building and Quebec nationalism), at the same time that it attempted to increase the degree of certainty in its budgetary environment. Then, in 1982 the federal government applied the reduced EPF escalator to the entire transfer, which meant that the provinces suffered from budgeting uncertainty caused by federal fiscal restraint. In the meantime, the federal budget deficit was growing.[26]

By 1990 most provincial governments had devised reform strategies to respond to the increasing uncertainty that had an impact on all policy areas, but affected health care in particular because of the large proportion of expenditure budgets devoted to this sector. In addition, the rapid advancement of medical technology and the aging of the population meant that health care costs continued to rise in spite of cutbacks. In 1995 the federal government announced that EPF and the Canada Assistance Plan (CAP) would be amalgamated into a single transfer: the Canada Health and Social Transfer (CHST). This reduced the total transfer for health, post-secondary education, and social assistance by approximately $6 billion,[27] generating further uncertainty in this area.

In the early stages of this period of retrenchment, governments were careful not to alarm the citizenry. Somehow it had to appear that social rights were being protected within the environment of cost containment. Hence, expectations had to be reshaped or replaced with more appealing prospects to address and reverse the trend of widening disjunction between the benefits and burdens of citizenship. Citizens felt entitled to a comprehensive range of health services, provided in decent facilities by competent caregivers within a reasonable amount of time, not just because they believed that the state ought to provide such benefits, but because they had already paid for them through their taxes. However, citizens' corresponding belief that the universal health system was a matter of national identity, transformed the social program into an important political symbol, which was effective as a constraint to change. This proved to be particularly frustrating for politicians, public servants, and practitioners, and virtually all people concerned agreed that the system needed to be reformed, although there was no consensus on *how* it should be reformed.

Changed Expectations: The New Language of Rights

As briefly noted already, the right to health care in the 1940s translated as the expectation that communicable diseases and other public health issues would be brought under control, and that a range of advanced medical services would be available in Canada for private consumption. Then in the 1950s and 1960s, with federal action in the policy field, the right to health care began to indicate an expectation that hospital and medical services would be distributed as public goods. Health care as social right was essential for the prosperity of the country and the abatement of social class. By the end of the next decade, health care had become part of Canada's collective conscience and protecting the right against retrenchment was a matter of practical concern, as well as national identity. In the 1980s, three major (and mutually reinforcing) forces commenced and gained momentum in Canada, which, in combination, explain the pursuant change in rights culture. The first is the rhetoric of the 'marketization of the state.' The second is the dual emphasis on individual/legal rights and collective identities that is the legacy of the 1982 Charter of Rights and Freedoms. The third is the Canada Health Act (1984) that asserted the role of the state in the health care arena.

There are, at least, two dynamics to observe in regard to the 'shift.' First, expectations were already high, and increasing in response to retrenchment and perceived threats to social entitlement. With each of the three 'forces' noted above, there was a discernible change in expectations. Second, the form of the rights claims changed. That is, distinct from the change in expectations, there was a change in acuity of intentions. For example, it seems that instead of rights claims indicating that the state should provide publicly the benefits of medical advancements to the entire Canadian population (as was the case in the 1960s), they have come to indicate that, by virtue of consumer power or as a matter of individual legal compensation, citizens are entitled to services because they have purchased them in advance, or they simply have legitimate and legally enforceable claims against the state.

Explaining the Shift in Rights Culture: Expectations and Intentions

The first factor in the trend is the decline of the citizen *as citizen* and the rise of the citizen as client or consumer of public services. This shift is part of a larger international trend that has been identified as the 'marketization of the state.'[28] Jon Pierre states:

> Politics and markets appear so far to be just as intertwined as they were in the 1960s and 1970s, only with the important difference that this time it is the market philosophy dominating politics, not the other way around as was previously the case. Along with the 'rolling back of the state' there evolved a 'vacuum' with regard to the rights of individuals; as the material elements of citizenship were abolished or transformed into services provided under private auspices, citizenship had to be redefined and reaffirmed. Moreover, since such a reaffirmation of the individual in relationship to the state was at the heart of the individualistic culture which characterized the 1980s, there were a number of different political forces pulling in the same direction.[29]

One result of this convergence of forces is the redefinition of Canadian social citizenship. This redefinition is particularly interesting in the case of health care because the politics–markets relationship seems to be reversed, which gives health care a great level of immunity against market forces. As Patricia O'Reilly explains, 'now [with the development of public health insurance], rather than being another economic market sector with social side-effects, health policy became a social policy sector with economic side-effects.'[30] However, retrenchment in health care seemed to be inevitable given the fiscal situation (marked by uncertainty and scarcity), and citizens began to assert their rights to health services with new meaning and unprecedented conviction.

To achieve quiescence in the face of reform efforts, which amounted to perceived rights violations, governments offered 'client' or 'consumer' status to a less deferential populace. The 'political empowerment' that was conferred through social rights was being replaced with 'economic empowerment.'[31] This changed the nature of the citizen–state exchange process from a traditional model of exchange based on 'needs, obligations and entitlements, with a market-like exchange process. In this [latter] exchange process, service providers under different auspices are assumed to be in competition with each other. Customers choose in a rational fashion between different service providers, thus sending signals regarding the quality of different services.'[32] This conception has not been fully institutionalized in Canada, although its limited appearances (mostly in the language of policy proposals and documents) likely influenced citizens' expectations.

The rhetoric of the new public management contributed to the redefinition of citizenship. In theory, the much sought after efficiency that is assumed to be generated by private market-type processes becomes the goal of governance. To achieve this goal, changes are made to the management structures of public organizations, and an ethic of customer service replaces the ethic of entitlement. In the process, 'rights' become service standards.

In Great Britain, for example, a Patient's Charter was drafted to inform National Health Service (NHS) clients that they were entitled to health services provided according to specified criteria (such as maximum waiting times), and that there were options for recourse in the event that the criteria were not met. Changes to the structure of the NHS in Britain were extensive: a system of 'managed competition' was devised to maximize efficiency in the provision of health services. This included the designation of certain fundholding general practitioners to manage budgets for all NHS general practitioners in a given area.

In Canada, changes to the management of health systems were not as extensive. However, the rhetoric of change in public management, as well as initiatives for structural change, gave the appearance that government was working hard to get the budget under control at the same time that it was making necessary improvements to the health care system.

Coincident with this declining trend is the frequent complaint that citizens have paid for health services in advance through their taxes, and therefore ought to be able to use those prepaid benefits when need arises. The expectation, then, is that of a simple market-type exchange of money (taxes) for services (health care). The intention, or course of action open to patients who feel that this exchange has not been completed, is unclear. It is not always possible for citizens to 'exit' from the relationship and seek to exchange money for benefits elsewhere. Of course, it is impossible for citizens to exit from the obligation of paying taxes.

The second factor is the new conception(s) of rights that emerged with the Charter of Rights and Freedoms. There is no consensus on the question of whether the Charter privileges the rights of individuals or groups. According to Raymond Bazowski, 'by endorsing affirmative action programs ... the Charter has paved the way for yet another concept of equality to emerge in the contemporary Canadian political vocabulary – equality of groups.'[33] However, the degree to which the Charter promotes 'affirmative action programs,' and hence group rights, is highly debatable. The Charter does not contain any substantive public policy prescriptions. On the contrary, the Charter promotes a 'procedural view of justice in which the commitment to treat all individuals equally and fairly takes precedence over any substantive shared end a society might favour.'[34] In other words, the Charter is primarily about legal procedure in which the possessive (property) rights of individuals take precedence over other conceptions of right. Reg Whitaker is unequivocal in his assessment: 'certainly it is self-evident that a dominant rights-based discourse is tied logically to the leading role of the courts in defining the boundaries of rights and defining many of the public policy implications of these rights.'[35] Again, the Charter is correctly identified as a procedural document, in which the rights possessed by individuals are codified. Hence, the Charter represents a departure from, and therefore an indirect attack on, the normative conception of right that defines social rights. What ought to be done (by society, for society)? is replaced with: What constitutes an illegal infringement on the moral space of an individual?

Quite clearly, it is the intentions of claiming rights that have changed. Although there are only a few well-documented cases of health care litigation (for instance, claims filed by persons who contracted HIV/AIDS or hepatitis C through tainted blood, the case brought against hospitals in British Columbia in regard to access to sign-language interpreters for hearing-impaired patients,[36] and the 'Charter challenge to the Nova Scotia government's decision not to fund a particular in vitro fertilization service known as ICSI'[37]), it is likely that the courts will be increasingly involved in important decisions concerning distributional equity in health care. So, even if expectations remain the same (expectations of hearing-impaired patients to have full access to care), the form or intention of the claim has changed; it can now be reinforced with legal action.

This is problematic because it means that citizens' legal–constitutional rights will increasingly come into conflict with ethical–medical issues. The ethic of informed consent, for instance, was overridden in a 1986 Charter case. Marcia Rioux explains that 'the case concerned the sterilisation of a young woman who could not give informed consent, and the court ruled that consent was not the issue. What mattered was the fundamental right of a woman to be able to bear children.'[38] In another case, an Alberta man with Down syndrome was denied an organ transplant. 'He was finally considered for a transplant as a result of public pressure, but by then it was too late and he had died.'[39] Rioux explains that in the past, such decisions were made by 'health providers alone.' Greater transparency and inclusiveness in decision-making, in addition to an almost dogmatic regard for individual rights, completely change the ways in which medical and bioethical issues are dealt with in the Canadian health system. In Rioux's estimation, this will lead ultimately to better legal and ethical standards.[40] However, this individual rights focus will still need to be reconciled with epidemiological evidence that indicates patterns of health and disease are linked to the ascribed, socioeconomic, and environmental conditions of communities.

As explained, the changes effected by the Charter's dual commitments impacted both individuals and groups. The post–Charter era in Canada is marked by attempts to recognize the rights of the latter without diminishing those of the former. Will Kymlicka and Wayne Norman thoroughly explain the most recent challenge to social rights:

> Marshall saw citizenship as a shared identity that would integrate previously excluded groups within British society, and provide a source of national unity. He was particularly concerned to integrate the working classes, whose lack of education and economic resources excluded them from the 'common culture' which should have been a 'common possession and heritage.'
>
> It has become clear, however, that many groups – Blacks, women, aboriginal peoples, ethnic and religious minorities, gays and lesbians – still feel excluded from the 'common culture,' despite possessing the common rights of citizenship. Members of these groups feel excluded, not only because of their socio-economic status, but also because of their socio-cultural identity – their difference.[41]

Health status maps onto cultural status in many instances. Insofar as recognition for multicultural claims is reflected in identity, that identity is constructed on the basis of inequality. While there might be something authentic expressed in 'culture,' the recognition of that authenticity is a form of political compensation. Groups that are not marginalized are not candidates for recognition. Groups that are marginalized because their cultural integrity has been devalued, experience other, predictable forms of social inequality, such as differences in health (both health status and access to services). Health, therefore, is relevant to identity; everyone has a health status, and that health status intersects with culture, lifestyle, and social class. The promise of equality (sameness of status) from universally available social programs, is somewhat dated in the context of differentiated citizenship. If the social rights thesis is outmoded, what are the implications for the right to health care in Canada?

Paradoxically, the institutionalization of the symbolic value of health care is beneficial in that it protects the right to health care (i.e., the existing, universal distribution of health care services), but problematic in that it perpetuates old models of care (e.g., medical and institutional), at a time when new approaches need to be considered (such as preventive medicine, recognition of social determinants of health, deinstitutionalization and home or community-based care). Furthermore, continued, uncritical defences of the right to health care are co-incident with the marginal erosion of the health system. In their reluctance to explicitly ration health services, governments ration on the margins by delisting some medical procedures and moving patients from hospital to un- or under-funded home care settings, without implementing new policies or providing resources to support the changes.

In response to pressing issues of cost, access, and accountability, the federal government introduced the 1984 Canada Health Act (CHA). The primary purpose of the legislation was to assert the role of the state in health care, especially that of the federal government as defender of Canada's sacred trust. The act specified conditions of payment upon which transfers would continue to be disbursed to the provinces (initially iterated in the Established Programs Financing arrangements), and, more importantly, the penalties that would be exacted for contravention of the act. Such penalties were intended to discontinue the practice of extra-billing by physicians, which constituted a symbolic disparagement of the state's commitment to universal health care (rather than a serious threat to public access).[42]

The degree to which the CHA heightened expectations is debatable. The five stated conditions of payment, comprehensiveness, accessibility, portability, universality, and public administration, are commonly, and somewhat incorrectly, referred to as 'principles' of medicare. Such misrepresentation might indicate that the CHA should represent higher goals, or fundamental precepts. The CHA does embody the stated goals of the federal government. But the authority of the act is connected to the financial penalties, not to the 'rightness' of moral assertions.

The CHA is important because it establishes the federal government's role in health care, which is a field of exclusive provincial jurisdiction. The act is also a source of stasis. As Raisa Deber explains, the CHA effectively regulates the provision of care in hospitals and other institutional settings delivered by physicians and surgeons.[43] Thus, any care delivered outside of this arrangement is not regulated by the act, and not within the purview of the federal government. Home care programs, for example, are being implemented in many provinces in response to the needs of patients – advancements in medical technology and pharmaceuticals make unnecessary many traditional patterns of health service delivery. However, home care options are not publicly funded (although they are, in some cases, subsidized according to means). The pharmaceuticals that make possible the delivery of care in the community are also outside the boundaries of most public plans. As Deber makes clear:

> The national terms [of the Canada Health Act] require the provinces to provide for all medically necessary physician and hospital services, without co-payments to insured persons for insured services. But this restriction to the services covered under the previous legislation is becoming increasingly outdated. As technology allows us to provide care in the community, the rhetoric of reformers bumps up against the uncomfortable fact that moving care away from physicians and hospitals also moves it outside of the jurisdiction of the Canada Health Act. Any services outside the Act can be deinsured.
>
> For this reason, the pharmacare and homecare programs now being called for do not represent frills. Canada is increasingly using the move to the community to privatize the financing of care.[44]

Clearly, there needs to be greater diversity and flexibility in health care service delivery. However, whatever changes are made, decision-making authority should continue to rest primarily with caregivers and the state. As already noted, the CHA makes arrangements for health care to be provided by medical doctors and practitioners in institutional settings. It might be advisable to change the language of the act so that 'medical doctors' are replaced with 'caregivers,' and then have the definition of 'caregiver' expanded in the act. Such a change might be effective in establishing viable home care programs. This suggestion recognizes the need to adjust the medical model (more will be said about this in Chapter 6) and the need to maintain stability and responsibility in fiscal federal arrangements.

Conclusion

The Charter's dual commitments to legal, procedural rights of the individual and categorical equity of historically marginalized groups demonstrate that citizenship in Canada requires constitutional respect for individual rights as well as group difference. Differences based on gender, sexual orientation, ethnicity, language, and ability, as they intersect with one another and socioeconomic status, demand recognition and accommodation, not strict equality. In the field of health care, flexibility is constrained by the institutionalization of health care as social right. While the importance of universality has not abated, the way in which universality is achieved (through preservation of the medical model and patterns of institutional care) is no longer entirely appropriate.

In the following chapter it is suggested that Canada has entered a fourth stage of citizenship development in which both collective and individual dimensions should be (and in some cases, already are) recognized. This development can be discerned in the parallel arguments concerning differentiated citizenship in general, and the right to health care in particular, which reveal the same patterns. To be clear, citizens' expectations or 'rights discourse' often do not reflect trends in health care provision, so much as they provide resistance to them. While the argument in this chapter has been that rights claims for health care have become more individualistic, health care continues to be distributed universally as a public good. When the collective assertions of right were made by the Canadian Federation of Agriculture, or Tommy Douglas, health services were delivered and funded privately. This gap between rights expectations and intentions is also explored in the next chapter.

4

The Right to Health Care

The Canadian health care system as a social policy experiment has proven to be a successful redistributive program. It is also a political symbol that distinguishes Canada from the United States, and as such transforms Canadian identity. Current changes in the system relating to patterns of deinstitutionalization, rising costs of pharmaceuticals, and the epidemiological contours of disease, in addition to the recognition that there might not be enough public money to meet demand, are causing health policy analysts to rethink the ways in which health services are funded and delivered.

On a more conceptual plane it can be observed that symbolic disputes over health care are no longer exclusively intergovernmental affairs, but involve citizens directly and evoke from them passionate responses in the language of rights. However, the terrain of social rights in Canada, of which the right to health care is a subset, is largely unfamiliar territory.[1] The social rights thesis, which provides the foundation for rights discourse in regard to social services, was advanced by British sociologist T.H. Marshall in 1949, and is not sophisticated enough to be relevant to current discussions of health care rights.[2] This makes necessary an examination of the meanings and significance of the right to health care within historical interpretations of right, as well as within contemporary conceptions of differentiated citizenship.

The 'right to health care' seems to have an inalienable collective dimension that is currently being challenged by possessive, individualistic rights claims. It is imperative to understand this collective dimension at this critical time in Canada's social policy history so that reform efforts will be channelled towards reconciling health care entitlement with differentiated conceptions of citizenship and away from litigious asseverations and actions. To this end, a conceptual model for health care can draw on recent investigations into the philosophical and political dynamics of cultural claims for recognition of identity and group rights.[3]

In this chapter, I am concerned mostly with the conceptual dimensions of the 'right to health care' debate. Canadians began asserting their rights to health care as early as the 1940s,[4] and now assert their rights with great frequency, albeit with different expectations and intentions. The first sections will examine the validity of rights, and the soundness of philosophical justifications for various conceptions of right. I argue that rights are important politically, in spite of their philosophical weaknesses. Building on this claim, in the following sections I try to determine the meaning of the right to health care by considering three possible conceptions of right, and proceed to argue that the right to health care has its roots in non-possessive, non–property-based rights, a conception that is in tension with current individualistic rights claims.

The Social Rights Thesis

Social citizenship, as conceived by Marshall, provides the basis for an explanation of the development of the right to health care in Canada. Marshall, in accepting the logic of capitalism, argues that the inequality of private markets ought to be offset with universally distributed social goods. Such redistribution will ensure equal substance of citizenship. In plain language, even though some citizens will be rich and others poor, there should be certain public goods to which all are entitled on equal terms and conditions. Otherwise, what it means to be a British citizen has no meaning independent of social class.

Despite the abundance of commentary on social rights, there is a profound lack of Canadian commentary on the subject.[5] This is surprising because health care in Canada is a perfect case study for social rights and citizenship theories. It might also be said that health care in Canada presents a puzzle. The right to health care is paradigmatic of Canadian culture, but is also an enigmatic social democratic covenant. Universal health care seems to be definitive of Canadian identity, while at the same time it presents a special case.[6] The pieces to this puzzle and the rights claims that defend it need further examination.

Rights Discourse

It is almost impossible to imagine political debate without the discussion of rights. In Canada, as in the United States, governments that enact legislation to ban smoking, limit public access to information, close a school, or increase restrictions on the possession of firearms have met with heavy resistance from their citizens. In almost every case, this resistance is expressed in the language of rights: 'I have the right to smoke.' 'I have the right to know what happened.' 'I have the right to send my children to the school of my choice.' 'I have the right to carry a gun.'

Some rights seem to be fundamental. Others seem to be frivolous, if indeed they are rights at all. Who decides what counts as a right? Surely, it cannot be the alleged bearer; there must be some internal logic to the idea of rights. It is critically important that this internal logic is deciphered now because, with the re-evaluation and reform of social programs, 'rights talk' in Canada has reached its high-water mark. People have come to believe that they have rights to the social goods that were provided by governments during the growth of the welfare state: namely, universal health care and publicly subsidized post-secondary education. It should come as no surprise that the political stakes are high for governments that make adjustments to these perceived rights. Citizens know that their rights are important, and that to be denied rights is to be denied something of great consequence, even though they rarely understand the implications of making rights claims. To determine what citizens mean when they talk about the right to health care, an adequate standard of living, or publicly subsidized university education, and whether they have such rights, it is necessary to sort through the 'rights talk' and establish the philosophical and political bases of rights.

What Is a Right?

To begin this undertaking, it is first necessary to determine exactly how rights are defined philosophically. Many such definitions are drawn from natural rights theories. H.L.A. Hart, in 'Are There Any Natural Rights?,' explains that if interference with the freedom of another person requires a moral justification, then it follows that there is at least one natural right, which is the equal right of all persons to be free.[7]

According to Hart, there is an 'essential connection between the notion of a right and the justified limitation of one person's freedom by another.'[8] What counts as a justified limitation? A limitation is justified, and hence a competing right, if it leads to a desirable distribution of human freedom.

The right of every person to be free constitutes *the* fundamental natural right because (1) it is plausible, if not self-evident, that all persons capable of (rational) choice can possess this right, and (2) this right is not 'created or conferred by men's voluntary action; other moral rights are.'[9] To have this natural right means that (a) all persons must refrain from exercising their freedom in the form of coercion, restraint, or harm against others, except to hinder coercion, restraint, or harm,[10] and (b) every person is at liberty to do any action that is not ruled out by (a). However, this foundational right is not unconditional or absolute. Constraints may be justified by special conditions, provided that they are consistent with the general principle of freedom. Consequently, Hart's position, as he admits, is not as ambitious as those of other natural rights theorists. But Hart defends his seemingly weak view by asserting that 'the principle that all men have an equal right to be free, meager as it may seem, is probably all that the political philosophers of the liberal tradition need to have claimed to support any program of action even if they claimed more.'[11] This is an acceptable and convincing philosophical justification for the idea of a right, but its weakness is that it raises more questions than it answers.

There are no definitive answers to such questions as: What counts as a justified limitation? If the answer to that question is that a limitation is justified if it leads to a proper or desirable distribution of human freedom, then it is immediately evident that there will be no agreement on what, exactly, 'proper or desirable' means and so on. Moreover, the term 'rights' is only a word that represents a code of moral behaviour, which, conceivably, is replaceable with other language. It may seem that the easiest course of action would be to dispense with talk about 'rights' altogether. However, rights are important political currency that cannot readily be discarded.

The Philosophical and Political Importance of Rights

The infungibility of rights is best demonstrated by Joel Feinberg's construction of a fictitious political community, 'Nowheresville,' where citizens have no rights. Feinberg directs us to: 'Try to imagine

Nowheresville – a world very much like our own except that no one, or hardly anyone (the qualification is not important), has *rights*.'[12] This exercise is immediately disturbing because it is counterintuitive; rights have become very important instruments for expressing political claims. Governments that deny their citizens rights in virtually any form are seen to be denying recognition of humanity, on the one hand, and political compensation for this recognition, on the other. Thus, Feinberg offers, if this 'flaw' (the absence of rights) makes Nowheresville too ugly a place to contemplate, it can be made more attractive with other moral features. For example, the concept of duty will exist in Nowheresville, but only in the weak sense of the term. In the strong sense, duty is associated with actions or goods that are owed someone, and is the correlative of a right. If Person A borrows money from Person B and promises to pay it back as soon as possible, then it can be said that Person B has a *right* to be repaid, and Person A has a *duty* to fulfil her promise. Alternatively, if each person has a right to free speech – a right in the strong sense, according to Ronald Dworkin, and one of a subset of rights to the right to freedom which, in Hart's view, is *the* fundamental human right – then each person also has a correlative duty not to interfere when others are expounding their views. However, in some cases, interference is necessary. People are prohibited from making defamatory remarks about others and from making comments that incite hatred against particular people or groups of people in society ('fighting words'). These restrictions constitute rights in that they are moral justifications for interference with the freedom of others.[13] This interference counts as a legitimate justification because it leads to a proper distribution of human freedom; by limiting the freedom of racists to say what they think, the freedom of members of minority groups is protected.

In Nowheresville this strong notion of duty is absent. What is allowed instead is a paler version of the term, one that indicates morally required action. Feinberg gives the example of a man who gives away his entire supply of poison to other prisoners so that they can commit suicide (in order to escape 'the burning alive that was to be their fate and his).[14] This man surely did not think that the other prisoners had more of a right to it than he did, although he felt morally obligated (that he had a duty in the weaker sense of the term) to give it to them.

Nowheresville is generally a very pleasant place where people respect the law. The 'moral practices' of personal desert and a sovereign rights monopoly are also included. The latter refers to a situation in which people have obligations not to each other, but to God or a sovereign. For every type of right that exists in the real world, there is a moral practice that replaces it in Nowheresville. When rights are excluded from political discourse, however, something of great importance is lost.

Repudiating Rights Talk

In contradistinction to Feinberg, Robert Young suggests that human rights talk should be substituted with moral 'ought talk' (the recognition of moral principles without possessive rights claims).[15] Young believes that the only valid conceptions of rights are those of legal rights and judgments that are formed on the basis of correct moral principles. This means that it is unintelligible to say that human rights are being violated in China or the United States, for example. Rather, in the language of 'ought talk,' we should say that 'the government of China *ought* to recognize the sovereignty of its citizens,' or 'the Chinese government *ought* not to arbitrarily arrest and detain its citizens,' or 'the United States government *ought* not to execute its citizen-felons.' These claims are so feebly stated that they seem somewhat absurd. Referring to these abuses as human rights violations strengthens the moral claim and signifies that much is at stake. In each case, the problem is not that a government, or governments, or a community ought to do a certain action, or ought not to continue another, but that fundamental rights are being violated – rights that should be recognized so that they are placed well beyond the whim of any individual, group or government.

In the case of health care, as will be explained, the right to services is a second-order human right and, as such, is accurately translated with an ought statement. That citizens have the right to health care does translate as 'the state ought to provide health services to all of its citizens.' However, as demonstrated in the examples of first-order human rights, the language of rights has great political impact in spite of the philosophical shakiness of the claims.

The deficiencies of Nowheresville and moral 'ought talk' are numerous and fundamental. As Feinberg notes, the making of moral claims (which would include both first- and second-order human rights) is essential to what it means to be human. Hence, the absence of rights represents the denial of the human character in political society. Feinberg explains this last point very well:

Having rights enables us to 'stand up like men [and women],' to look others in the eye, and to feel in some fundamental way the equal of anyone. To think of oneself as the holder of rights is not to be unduly but properly proud, to have that minimal self-respect that is necessary to be worthy of the love and esteem of others. Indeed, respect for persons (this is an intriguing idea) may simply be respect for their rights, so that there cannot be the one without the other; and what is called 'human dignity' may simply be the recognizable capacity to assert claims. To respect a person then, or to think of him as possessed of human dignity, simply *is* to think of him as a potential maker of claims. Not all of this can be packed into a definition of 'rights'; but these are *facts* about the possession of rights that argue well their supreme moral importance. More than anything else I am going to say, these facts explain what is wrong with Nowheresville.[16]

While Nowheresville is clearly deficient, as described, Feinberg's justification of rights is convincing, yet philosophically flimsy. It is not clear that the idea of a right has a solid philosophical grounding. What Feinberg's explanation suggests is that rights are significant because they protect individual dignity and autonomy at the same time that they connect all human beings in 'some fundamental way.' That rights can, and do, embody this duality is extraordinary and demonstrates their indispensability. This does not, however, fully explain why rights have become so important in everyday discussions in recent years. Why are people always talking about their rights?

As indicated, part of the answer is that the political justifications for the idea of a right are quite strong in spite of the philosophical precariousness of the term. First of all, the term 'right' enables a discussion of moral practices without the moral label. In modern political life it seems that the state is considered to be a *neutral* guarantor and protector of rights,[17] and therefore not a legitimate participant in debate over morals. Second, rights guarantee individual autonomy. In Nowheresville, or a world in which human rights talk has been replaced with moral 'ought talk,' human beings are dependent on the benevolence of a sovereign for formulations of the 'good society.' Third, rights have come to define what is justly expected from governments and from other citizens. The other part of the answer is that the idea of rights is rooted in certain historical developments that are essential to modern morality. Both possible answers will be considered more thoroughly with the discussion of social rights and health care entitlement in the following sections.

The Historical Evolution of Rights: Three Conceptions

There are at least three meanings of 'right,' according to which social rights (and, as a subset of social right, the right to health care) can be evaluated. The first is that of 'human rights' which Dworkin calls rights in the 'strong sense.'[18] Rights in the strong sense, or first-order human rights, are argued to be prior to governments or political communities, and therefore not alterable (without strong moral justifications) by either.

The second conception is that of human rights in the weak sense, linked to the normative/objective *ius* of early Roman law. Richard Tuck[19] explains that 'right' (*ius*) was originally distinct from 'property' (*dominium*). 'Right' had a normative meaning that did not refer to the moral space (i.e., property) of individuals. The early Romans used the term within the context of divine judgment to define the way in which disputants in a trial ought to behave towards one another:

> Disputants took oaths as to the righteousness of their claims, one of which was upheld in a subsequent ordeal or other supernatural judgment. The favourable verdict was a *ius*. This is a significant origin in two ways. First, it shows that a *ius* was taken to be something objectively right and discoverable, and in this sense it remained as a kind of synonym for 'law' throughout the history of Latin as an effective language ... But the early use of the term *ius* also shows that it was generally taken to be the right way in which two disputants should behave towards each other, and did not (for example) cover criminal matters.[20]

This conception of right is relevant to the discussion of the right to health care because it reveals a 'third way' between human rights and legal rights (discussed below). The tangible benefits of universal health care provision and claims for that provision are grounded in a strong, non-possessive, normative argument. We might want to argue neither that the inability of the U.S. government to provide universal health care to its citizens constitutes a human rights violation, nor that barriers to health care access are merely legal matters. Like the *ius* that normatively determined how disputants in Rome ought to behave towards one another, social rights define how citizens ought to treat one another and what ought to be provided for them by the state.

In contemporary terms, this conception of human rights in the weak sense indicates that a person has a right to act according to his or her conscience or, as a subset of this, each person has a right to refuse to be drafted into the armed forces, or to refuse to pay illegitimate taxes. For example, I know of an American woman who did not want any of the money that she contributed through income taxes to be used to support the U.S. military. So she hired an accountant to determine what proportion of her taxes would go to the defence budget, and then she withheld that amount. She felt that she had the right to do this in that she felt morally obligated to act in accordance with her beliefs. In each of these cases it is clear that fundamental or human rights are not being exercised, or violated, to justify action, and that each action is explicitly prohibited by law. Rather, these cases involve consideration of 'doing the right thing,' or a normative evaluation of what ought to be done. As such, it is this conception that provides the basis for social rights. The view that all Canadian citizens are entitled to health care services provided on an equal basis is grounded in the belief that it is morally right to do so, that it is morally right to provide less fortunate people with equal benefits.

The third conception is the right to health care as a legal right. Throughout this book I argue that rights claims for health care are increasingly legalistic in nature. When citizens claim that they have the right to health care, they have two intentions. The first is to assert their expectations, and the second is to back up their claim with legal force (even if this force is only rhetorical, and does not precipitate any litigious action). In short, there are two points to observe about contemporary health care rights claims. First, citizens' expectations seem to be consistent over time. The incremental nature of their expectations reflects past experiences and patterns of entitlement, as well as future entitlements to advanced medical technology, pharmaceuticals, and services. Second, the legalistic, individualistic force of the claims, as the result of changing political, economic, and social circumstances, impairs the possibility for much-needed improvements in the health care system because it is employed to reinforce or protect a rather rigid set of expectations.

Social Rights as Compensation

The theoretical validity of the second conception of right is reinforced by the arguments of Arthur Dyck and Thomas Paine. Dyck's general assessment of right is useful as a point of departure. Dyck claims: 'A right, then, is first and foremost a just expectation, that is, a state of being characterized by ties of mutually expected responsibilities to one another, as individuals and as members of groups and institutions.'[21] This definition seems to capture quite accurately what is being expressed when citizens claim that they have rights to universal health care, heavily subsidized post-secondary education, adequate levels of welfare assistance, and the like. 'I have the right to health care' can be translated as 'I justly expect that the state will provide the social goods that are necessary to guarantee an adequate standard of living to members of my political community.'

However, citizens' expectations have changed regarding health care as the epidemiological contours of disease have changed,[22] advanced medical technology has become available, and other components of the state–society relationship have been altered. Thus, the general statement that rights constitute just expectations, is, in itself, insufficient as a means of understanding contemporary rights claims. To fully comprehend the evolution of social rights as citizenship in Canada, there needs to be thorough examination of citizens' expectations and a more precise definition of the right to health care and the form that rights claiming takes.

A compelling definition is offered by Paine, who makes an argument for social rights as compensation in a 'little essay' entitled 'Agrarian Justice.' Paine explains that because poverty does not exist in a natural state, the first principle of civilization ought to be: 'That the condition of every person born into the world, after a state of civilization commences, ought not to be worse off than if he had been born before that period.'[23] According to Paine, every person born into the world has certain property rights. These are rights of usage – for example, the right to chop down a tree for wood to burn, to hunt animals for food, and to pick apples from trees, which exist because God gave the Earth to humans in common. The institution of private property has thereby 'dispossessed' some people of these natural property rights. Paine's proposed solution to this problem is

> to create a National Fund, out of which there shall be paid to every person, when arrived at the age of twenty-one years, the sum of fifteen pounds sterling, as a compensation in part, for the loss of his or her natural inheritance, by the introduction of the system of landed property: And also, the sum of ten pounds per annum, during life, to every person now living of the age of fifty years, and to all others as they shall arrive at that age.[24]

This redistribution scheme reflects the view that for a person to acquire personal property, the cooperation of others is required: 'All accumulation, therefore, of personal property beyond what a man's own hands can produce, is derived to him by living in society; and he owes on every principle of justice, of gratitude, and of civilization, a part of that accumulation back again to society from whence the whole came.'[25]

Because the institution of private property has caused some people to be relatively disadvantaged in that they cannot adequately provide for themselves, a supplementary set of rights to ensure substantive equality in society is required. The state has an obligation, as do all members of society (via taxes rather than charity), to guarantee a minimum standard of living to all its citizens, which in contemporary terms includes health care, education, and income assistance benefits. States that do not provide such rights to their citizens fail to recognize the nature of the dispossession that Paine describes, and thereby deny their citizens important benefits to which they are entitled.

As indicated, Paine's argument can be considered to be an early formulation of the social rights thesis, which was not popularized until the mid-twentieth century. For Paine, welfare entitlements are required as compensation for the violation of natural (individual) property rights. This conceptualization is rooted in the ideas of 'possessive individualism'[26] (property-based rights), which came to replace earlier, normative notions of right. Michael Hayes and Sholom Glouberman explain that 'in both health and development, we have experienced a shift from a pre-modern notion of collectivity to an Enlightenment sensibility of the rational individual as separate from nature.'[27] However, normative, non–property-based, collective dimensions still seem to account for some of the vagaries of social rights discourse.

Between Tuck and Paine: *Ius* versus *Dominium*

The general trend, for approximately the past 600 years, has been towards property-based, individual rights (*dominium*). Twentieth-century social rights seem to be an anomaly in that the original normative meaning of right (*ius*) is manifest in their conception. In Canada, until approximately 1980, there seemed to be conceptual equilibrium between *ius* and *dominium*. The right to health care was (perhaps inadvertently) conceived as a collective entitlement, definitive of Canadian citizenship, at the same time that it indicated an area of individual entitlement.[28] However, the changes effected by trends in public management reform that recast the citizen as a consumer or client of public services and introduce market mechanisms into public service delivery, and, more significantly, the Charter of Rights and Freedoms and the Canada Health Act, redefined the meaning of rights claims for access to health care. The nature of rights claims in the 1980s became more individualistic and legalistic. As perceived entitlements were challenged, and in some cases rescinded, in this period of increased legal–constitutional and consumer rights, Canadian citizens responded in kind. Citizens seem to have come to feel entitled to health services, and the (inevitable) rationing of services is perceived as a violation of rights. The right to health care is no longer merely a 'just expectation' or normative claim, but a serious legal matter.

How does this analysis fit with differentiated citizenship claims? Such claims are both possessive and normative. This means that they depart from modern, individualistic, possessive conceptions of right to embody historical patterns of marginalization, contingency, and identity. Thus, they are postmodern in that they have recaptured and recognized many premodern elements and rejected the abstract rationality of individual moral space as the basis for equality, freedom, and unity. However, differentiated citizenship claims are constructed within the framework of modernism, which is to say that they have retained commitments to rights, equality, and citizenship. The main point of departure is this: these claims pertain to groups, not individuals. The fruits of modernism are distributed to different groups with various identities, histories, needs, and preferences.

The conceptual configuration of differentiated citizenship claims, or identity rights, is similar to the conceptual configuration of social rights. As explained, social rights are rooted in communal notions of entitlement and normative rather than possessive conceptions of right. Social rights, as conceived by Marshall, are individualistic (in the way that Paine describes), possessive (but not tantamount to human rights), deontological (but not in the Kantian sense), and normative (which connects them to their early Roman legal roots). Therefore, the transformation of social rights throughout the centuries has become more individualistic and possessive, yet the enduring normative element harbours collectivist ideals. In this regard, social rights are conceptually similar to identity rights. Of course, social rights, as currently constituted, do not embody the idea that social goods will be distributed differentially, according to identity or other criteria. Social rights by definition are universal. By reconfiguring universality to reflect difference (in the way that the goal of 'equality' is understood to be achieved by recognizing and accommodating different capacities and circumstances of individuals), identity rights might be the next 'logical' step from Marshall's trinity. Such a step might be preferable to the legal rights orientation that is emerging in the health care arena in Canada.

Conclusion

The philosophical basis of a right, as either a justification for interference with the freedom of another person, a valid claim, or a just expectation, is quite weak despite the popularity of rights talk. The impact of asserting rights is political, and it is reinforced by governments trying to allocate moral, social, and economic resources to individuals. To discuss the philosophical and political bases of rights is to bring to the table the entire debate concerning the role of government; disagreement over moral rights parallels disagreement over the responsibilities of the state.

The non-possessive, normative nature of the 'right to health care' is a significant philosophical finding, one that informs the political debate over health care by revealing that current legal rights claims are not sufficient to defend social entitlements. Canadian citizens' expectations have changed incrementally since the 1940s, and have come to outpace governments' ability to provide access to health services. This gap between expectations and public capacity is a serious problem to which there is no easy solution.

The purpose of explaining this change in rights discourse as it pertains to rights claiming for access to health services is not merely to engage in hand wringing over the individualistic and legalistic attack on the 'good old days' of community-based norms of social citizenship. Rather, the point is to evaluate the evolving meaning and substance of the right to health care in Canada. Marshall himself would encourage revision in the context of new social, political, and economic dynamics. What direction will citizenship development take in the twenty-first century?

5

Sources of Stasis: Budgeting, Perceptions of Privatization, and the Politics of Federalism

In Chapters 2 and 3 I explained that the social rights thesis was outdated. In this chapter I argue that the changing dynamics of citizenship, in addition to the effects of a post-Keynesian, global economy, altered the substance of social rights. Also, I will consider the implications of the institutionalization of the right to health care in Canada, and argue that social rights stasis is reinforced by citizens' resistance to the commodification of health services and the politics of federalism. This will serve as a more empirical response to the conceptual question that was considered in the previous chapter.

Stasis is problematic because it precludes adoption of more appropriate models of care. Paradoxically, defences of social rights, as originally formulated, reinforce the medical model at the same time that they recognize the need for change in the system. As noted in a preceding chapter, social rights hold constant the mechanics of the health care system. The principles and logic of the system, not caused by social rights but defined by them, are dependent on stable patterns of public finance and service provision. Thus, reluctance to question social rights seems to translate as reluctance to question the institutional logic of the system.

The problems presented by stasis reach well beyond intergovernmental discord and symbolic disparagement. If the current situation continues, with or without additional public funding, health care will deteriorate. As the World Health Organization reports, 'a clear historical lesson emerges from health systems development in the twentieth century: spontaneous, unmanaged growth in any country's health system cannot be relied upon to ensure that the greatest health needs are met.'[1] More deliberate and integrative approaches to reform are needed.[2] The epidemiological transition, thoroughly explained in Chapter 6, defines the shift in main causes of disease and death from communicable to non-communicable diseases. The noting of such a shift is important not only because it effectively indicates the changing contours of disease, but because those contours reveal new dynamics of citizenship. Policy responses are needed to address the epidemiological transition and pressures for growth.

Sources of Stasis

Issues of entitlement in health care are becoming, simultaneously, more complex and more important. In the United States, inequitable patterns of access to health insurance, and hence services, are becoming sharper and more apparent as the managed care industry falters. Individuals who are not 'entitled' to health care, either through their jobs or government programs, are concerned about cost and quality of care. For approximately 44 million Americans with no insurance,[3] and for an even greater number whose insurance is meagre, with substantial co-pays, and contingent on employment, the question: what do I do if I (or my kids, or parents, or spouse) get sick? is engulfing.

To borrow again from the U.S. experience, changing notions about the omnipotence of medicine adds to the complexity of health care issues. In the 1970s in the United States the development of Health Maintenance Organizations (HMOs), in addition to the engagement of communities in decision-making exercises, challenged the autonomy of physicians. The situation today is such that corporate control of medicine gives the appearance, at the very least, that doctors' hands are tied in decision-making, and care is dependent on cost feasibility.[4]

In Canada there are discernible cracks in the universality of health care provision. In most cases, pharmaceuticals are outside the purview of public plans, and, as such, there are 'communities' of affected persons with spurious and indefinite entitlements. In Canada, although there is complicated interprovincial variation in patterns of entitlement for expensive drugs, it is unlikely that many will have to declare bankruptcy in an effort to maintain their health. However, the entitlement issue becomes the availability of care, regardless of costs.

The Canadian health system is usually examined along two axes. The more common, that of federalism, and the counterpoint, medical profession–state accommodation, are examined carefully in relation to one another by Carolyn Hughes Tuohy, who argues that the latter is the better explanatory axis.[6] Tuohy's work is convincing and more sophisticated than the litany coming from scholars who favour the former. Miriam Smith (as a proponent of federalism as the primary explanatory axis), for example, argues that 'the combination of parliamentary governance and the particular features of federal arrangements in medicare increases the federal government's scope for unilateral retrenchment in the medicare field.'[7] This only scratches the surface. What pushes the intergovernmental agenda? What are the details in the big picture?

Tuohy submits that the truth in the details can be discerned in the dynamics of the politics of the medical profession. In brief, the monopolist position (organized medicine) has been stronger than that of the monopsonist (government), because 'the state developed a "second-level" agency relationship with the profession, which acknowledged the primacy of professional judgment.'[8] However, with the extra-billing issue in the 1970s and 1980s, for the first time, organized medicine failed to win major concessions from the state, in part because citizens' expectations did not permit concession.

Tuohy points out in her book *Accidental Logics*, 'In the 1990s, the state sought both to reduce sharply the rates of increase in public spending and to substantially extend the terms of its accommodation with the profession. In so doing, it placed great strain on the profession-state relationship and on the ability of the profession to manage the complex internal balances upon which that relationship depended.'[9]

However, there seems to be another important factor in the determination of health policy. In the case of governments reversing decisions to delist certain 'medically necessary services,'[10] it seems to have been public sentiment that was the main source of pressure, not physicians. Perhaps the Canada Health Act (1984) was less benign than is sometimes thought as it confirmed the entrenchment of social rights.[11] Citizens' expectations and entitlement have, therefore, challenged, at the very least, professional judgment and interests as the primary explanation for stability.

Tuohy's argument makes good sense, and covers both major axes, but does not directly address the linchpin issue. How can Tuohy explain patterns of medical profession – state accommodation without examining the 'just expectations' of citizens? Why would the state regularly make major concessions to the medical profession if citizens' expectations or social rights did not factor in?[12] Is it not the case that the citizenship bargain is at the foundation of interest group–government and intergovernmental disputes?

The Canadian Medical Association (CMA) is clearly influenced by public support for health care, as evidenced by the reluctance of the CMA in 1997 to go against the grain of public opinion and formally endorse a two-tiered system, as it was inclined to do. Of course, this is because it has its own agenda, not simply because it is benevolently interested in promoting social justice. The interests of organized medicine are served by the existing system, but the question remains, why do governments concede? Why is it in the interest of the state to protect the interests of the medical profession? Physicians are skilled at making it appear that threats to their autonomy are equal to infringements on entitlement.[13]

Furthermore, the fanfare surrounding Finance Minister Paul Martin's 1999 'health care budget,' signified in a very grand way that Canada had 'turned a corner,' had emerged from the era of retrenchment in health care, and that the federal government was prepared to bail the health care system out of its 'crisis.' The 1999 federal budget restored $11.5 billion to health care,[14] and the 2000 federal budget 'offered a one-time $2.5 billion fund to the provinces for health and education, which the provinces can draw down as they wish over the next five years.'[15] In September 2000, at the annual First Ministers Meeting, all provinces agreed to prepare annual health care report cards to ensure greater accountability in health care spending, and the federal government committed '$21 billion of additional cash through the CHST [Canada Health and Social Transfer] over the next five years, including $2.2 billion for Early Childhood Development.'[16] This was a welcome rapprochement in an otherwise turbulent and tense intergovernmental environment. To be sure, federalism is a constraint in its own right, but it is not driven by intergovernmental politics.

Intergovernmental disputes must have subtexts, wrangling must be directed at securing a political position. Those who say that federalism constrains change are not quite right. In effect, they argue that federalism causes intergovernmental tension, but that is disingenuous. It is certainly not an ambitious explanation: failing to explain why governments relentlessly quarrel over the issue of health care, it merely observes that they do.

The view of citizenship as it pertains to health care in Canada seems to be a much better (if elusive and mercurial) explanatory factor for governmental behaviour. Rights claiming does not seem to be wavering, and public support for universal health care continues to be strong, although Canadians are increasingly dissatisfied with the quality of the system. David Naylor reports that in a 1996 Gallup Poll almost 60 per cent of Canadians rejected the idea of two-tiered health care.[17] In an Angus Reid Poll conducted in May 2000, more than 50 per cent of all those surveyed listed health care as the highest priority presently confronting Canada.[18] In January 2000, approximately 25 per cent of all respondents rated the Canadian health care system as very good or excellent (in 1991 just over 60 per cent of respondents rated the system very good or excellent).[19] The challenge is for governments to notice and address the concerns of citizens and guide reform efforts accordingly.

Differentiated citizenship, is replacing the paradigm of universality and can be observed in health care politics. Communities of citizen–patients that fall outside traditional entitlement zones need representation and recognition that defences of the social rights thesis cannot accommodate. In short, social rights claiming influences patterns of behaviour of governments and organized interests. How the issue has not been addressed directly remains a mystery. Prominent scholars have hinted at it, but seem reluctant, perhaps for good reasons, to critique universal entitlement to health care.[20] Clearly, much is at stake.

My argument in this chapter proceeds as follows. Social rights claiming constrains change because (1) it does not reflect differentiation, but individual entitlement to a public good; (2) governmental decision-making seems to be subordinate to citizens' expectations. This is called democracy, and is not a completely negative arrangement. However, the citizenship 'bargain' prevents the system from reforming itself.

In this chapter sources of stasis are examined in order to develop the argument. There are four main sources of stasis, which make up the citizenship bargain: (1) budgeting, (2) perceptions of privatization, (3) the politics of federalism, and (4) organized medicine.

Privatization and the Politics of Federalism

Contributors to the health care debate who defend health care as a social right, or assert that health care is an important symbol of Canadian identity, often fail to realize that the symbolic value of health care and the politics of federalism are mutually reinforcing. That is, intergovernmental discord perpetuates the symbolic appeal of universal health care (federal and provincial governments both try to appear to be defenders of the 'sacred trust'), at the same time, the symbolic appeal of health care constrains political decision-making in the policy field. It is the latter dimension that requires further examination.

As noted, three factors serve to reinforce stasis by lending strength to defences of the social rights thesis. First, the justification for social rights made sense in the context of Keynesianism, relaxed scarcity in budgeting environments, and postwar nationalism, and has not been revised to take into account new trends. Second, there is heavy resistance of citizens to increased private sector involvement in health care.[21] This resistance limits the range of options available to governments to respond to the current financial situation. Third, decision-making is constrained by the politics of federalism; federal and provincial governments compete for the role of defender of citizens' rights to health care. More precisely, the federal government strives to maintain its moral authority in the health policy field by way of its constitutional spending power, and provincial governments blame the federal government for interfering in an area of provincial jurisdiction and for unilaterally reducing or determining federal spending commitments for health care (and thereby being responsible for provincial fiscal uncertainty). While this predicament might not be new or remarkable in nature, the context in which it is cast draws attention.

Redistributing Health Services

Health care reform in Canada, as a response to the widening gap between citizens' expectations and levels of service focuses on institutional rather than system change. The universal, single-payer model is not directly threatened by rational, comprehensive policy redirection, although it might be threatened indirectly by incremental, institutional changes. On the one hand, it seems that governments are maintaining a holding pattern to avoid making specific commitments for the future of the universal health care system. On the other hand, the nature of the issues involved (distributional, bioethical) precludes prompt and decisive action. Issues concerning the reallocation of health care resources and the replacement of medical and institutional models of care are not easily managed by governments, for several reasons, including the complexity of the issues involved, the degree of coordination required, and because citizens have come to regard health care as a right and an integral component of Canadian identity. Attempts to reduce or limit access to the health care system are considered to constitute rights violations.

At first glance, this seems to be a virtue. Governments must respect social rights and maintain political commitments to equity, regardless of their budgeting environments. However, political commitments also constrain much-needed changes. For example, evidence indicates there is increasing demand for alternative and complementary medicine,[22] yet physicians' services and hospitals consume the vast majority of resources.[23] However, when resources are redirected, and access to physicians is limited, or hospitals are closed, there is public outcry. The result is that rhetorical commitments are progressive and pay lip service to empowerment, preventive medicine, new approaches to care, and population health models, but political action is rendered static by the voracious symbolism of the right to health care.

What Is Stasis?

Carolyn Hughes Tuohy explains that the relative stability of the Canadian health care system, discernible in the context of pressurized budgeting and policy-making environments, presents a puzzle: 'Canada had, after all, one of the most expensive publicly funded health care systems in the world. Yet it experienced one of the lowest levels of institutional and structural change in the 1980s and 1990s.'[24] According to Tuohy, such stability can be attributed to the accommodation between the medical profession and the state. Even as the hospital share of total health care expenditure declined, there has been a relatively constant share of total health care expenditures distributed to physicians between 1975 and 1996.[25]

Stability in the distribution of expenditures for health care is supported by continued federal commitment to universal health care. The National Forum on Health (NFOH), appointed by the Chrétien government in 1994, tabled its report in 1997, which served to publicly reinforce the principles of the existing system.[26] The report of the NFOH, an almost exclusively federal document,[27] reasserted the 'key features' of the system – 'public funding for medically necessary services, the "single payer" model, the five principles of the Canada Health Act, and a strong federal/provincial/territorial partnership.'[28] However, the existing system was reaffirmed but not reassessed, so that the important recommendations made, regarding implementation of pharmacare and home care programs, and the creation of an ethics advisory committee, seemed to be options for additional services, not a new approach. As a result, the NFOH recommendations seemed to constitute a broad and hopeful agenda for the future, rather than a viable blueprint for change.

Although 'stasis' seems to be a pejorative term (relative to 'stability'), it is not simply an ideological locution that reflects disapproval of the status quo or planned restructuring in the social policy field. The traditional position of the left would be the defence of health care as a social right, not the repudiation of that assertion. To be clear, there are three indications of 'stasis,' as one step beyond 'stability.' The first indication of stasis is gridlock in federal provincial decision-making. For example, the reluctance of the federal government to critically reassess existing services and patterns of delivery, and to have proceeded with the exercise without support of the provinces, indicates the inadequacy of the NFOH exercise. It would seem that with the NFOH the federal government was effectively putting up resistance to provincial strategies for reform. Intergovernmental tension seemed to abate temporarily in September 2000, when all provinces agreed to greater scrutiny in their health spending (via report cards). However, with the appointment of the federal Commission on the Future of Health Care in Canada (chaired by Roy Romanow), provincial discord has resumed.

The second indication is policy reversals in response to public pressure. For example, in Ontario, the government's attempt to delist services that were not deemed medically necessary (beginning in 1993) was met with heavy public resistance. One of the most controversial items on the block was the annual health examination. The annual 'physical' provided little benefit, but in the end, was not removed from the list because it was 'premature pending the development of practice guidelines for preventive health care. It was also consistent with the government's own fears of the political ramifications of deinsuring such a commonly offered service.'[29] In Alberta, beginning in 1985, several procedures were delisted, such as family planning counselling, tubal ligations, vasectomies, and mammoplasty,[30] but many were eventually put back on the list because of public pressure. There are many other examples of policy reversals, or ambiguous policy commitments that are endemic to reform agendas. The most significant of the latter will be discussed in some detail in Chapter 7.

The third indication is stability in face of evidence of need for change. Changing demographics, new pharmaceuticals, deinstitutionalization, preventive medicine, advanced medical technology, and the epidemiological transition, all suggest that change is required. Yet the system is remarkably stable. Of course, stability in a turbulent policy field is advantageous. But in the case of health care, the complexity of issues and the importance of services, as well as the expense of the program, make it impossible that stability will prevail indefinitely, and that stability will be conducive to the type of development necessary to respond to current and future challenges.

What follows is a more detailed explanation of the sources of stasis that account for the lack of change in the health policy field (all of which are coincident with the entrenchment of the social right to health care), and, at the same time, indicate the need for change.

Budgeting for Health Care: The Changing Dynamics of Distribution

As the days of expanding public revenues begin to re-emerge in what has been termed the 'post-deficit' era, governments in North America continue to grapple with the complexities of budgeting in an uncertain and unstable environment. In the decades immediately following the Second World War, governments invested in the development of social programs. When economic growth declined, and fiscal restraint became necessary in the 1980s, governments ran deficit budgets in the hope that the economic times were merely temporary. However, by the 1990s, the situation was recognized to be unsustainable, and eliminating deficits and reducing debt became top priorities.

The effects of fiscal restraint in federal and provincial budgeting can be clearly discerned in health care, although this revered social program was shielded from cuts that befell other, less politically divisive, policy areas. In the period from 1991 to 1996, expenditures for health care declined (in real per capita terms) by approximately 5 per cent (total),[31] and the proportion of private expenditures increased,[32] although the Canadian Institute for Health Information and Statistics Canada report that the proportion of public expenditure is projected to rise.[33] Health care reform (and retrenchment) exercises were implemented at the margins of established programs, so that it would appear to citizens that their right to health care was being protected as governments worked to eliminate budget deficits.

In 1995, the federal government amalgamated funding for health and post-secondary education (Established Programs Financing) with the largest remaining shared-cost program (the Canada Assistance Plan) into a single transfer (the Canada Health and Social Transfer), which reduced federal financial commitments by approximately $6 billion over three years.[34] The position that governments would be able to protect health care despite fiscal 'crisis' had become untenable.

For the next three years (1995–8), provincial governments dealt unhappily with federal reductions in transfer payments. In many provinces, labour force contraction, de-insurance of 'medically unnecessary' procedures, and regionalization schemes were undertaken by governments as means of dealing with increased uncertainty in their own budgeting environments.

The 1999 federal budget looked like good news for all those concerned about erosion of the health care system. The promise of renewed funding had been fulfilled. With the elimination of its budget deficit, the federal government had committed $11.5 billion for reinvestment in health care,[35] to be disbursed to the provinces over the next five years. The 2000 federal budget provided a further $2.5 billion in cash, and the First Ministers Meeting in September 2000 the federal government allocated another $21.1 billion of additional cash through the CHST over the next five years.[36]

> This will bring the total cash transfer to the provinces and territories through the CHST to $18.3 billion in 2001–02, $19.1 billion in 2002–03, rising to $21.0 billion in 2005–06. In that year, CHST cash will be 35 per cent above the current level of $15.5 billion. Combined with the growth in the value of CHST tax points to $18.9 billion, the federal transfer to the provinces and territories will grow to $39.9 billion by 2005–06. To ensure further predictability, by the end of 2003–04, the federal government will establish the CHST cash transfers for years 2006–07 and 2007–08.[37]

In the context of changing demographics and the advancement of medical technology and new pharmaceuticals, this money is much needed. But it might not be sufficient to satisfy rising expectations. That is not to say that even stronger federal financial commitments are required to keep pace with demand, but that problems in the health care system run deeper than mere funding shortages.

The medical model of care is in need of re-evaluation, new medical equipment and drugs make institutional care increasingly unnecessary, and new patterns of inequality have been linked to health, all of which indicate the need for fundamental change. However, change is constrained by the institutionalization of health care as a social right of citizenship. Governments are reluctant to take any action that might be perceived as a threat to that right.

In short, the justification for social rights made more sense in the context of political commitments to Keynesianism, relaxed scarcity, and postwar nationalism, and is somewhat misplaced in budgeting environments marked by increasing numbers of competitive claims. The goal of governance in the 1990s has become respecting the diversity of these claims, not reducing them to a common denominator.

Economic Equilibrium Versus the Budget

According to John Maynard Keynes, whose economic doctrine guided North American economies during the postwar period of growth (1945–77), 'the goal of policy should be to balance not the budget, but the economy. The government should adopt the levels of spending, taxing, and borrowing that will produce acceptable levels of GNP, inflation and unemployment.'[38] At the same time, sociologist T.H. Marshall argued that the economy should be balanced by offsetting the inequalities generated by private markets with universal social programs.[39] Social rights, manifest in the creation of a universal health care system, are the products of economic equilibrium. The need to balance the economy, as indicated by Marshall, means that the distortions created by the economy (i.e., inequalities generated by capitalism) ought to be offset by recognizing social rights, and thereby guaranteeing social services as a matter of citizenship, rather than leaving social benefits to be determined by the market or other arbitrary forces.

The favourable economic conditions of the postwar period allowed governments to offer an expanded range of public services to their citizens. In many cases these increased resources were distributed as social programs, and responded directly to the demands placed on the state by rising expectations in a context of relative prosperity and technological advancement. A consequence was that citizens came to regard these new programs as entitlements, and so began a process of incremental 'ratcheting-up' of the resources to be distributed.[40] Entitlement programs, such as universal health care in Canada, and Medicare, Medicaid, and Social Security in the United States, came to be regarded as social rights of citizenship. They were more fully developed in Canada in part because, in the United States, the civil rights movement demanded the attention of governments and the courts and thereby diverted the focus from social rights to civil rights during this formative period.[41]

Governments in the 1990s struggled to eliminate budget deficits and lost sight of the need to 'balance the economy.' The need to address the importance of social rights in capitalist societies, the requirement for social safety nets to guard against economic adversity, or the proper distributions of the benefits and burdens of citizenship, are no longer considered; the economy is micro-managed to achieve the ultimate goal: a balanced budget. As Aaron Wildavsky and Naomi Caiden state, 'controlling the deficit has become a "metaphor for governing."'[42] But it does not make sense to suggest turning back the clocks. It has become clear that new complexities are not well accommodated within the context of the social rights paradigm. The social rights thesis, supported by political commitments to health care as a right of citizenship, needs to be revised, not simply defended.

The social vision of Keynesianism[43] had been replaced with more limited and immediate fiscal concerns, the impact of which was first felt in areas other than health care. Health care has been relatively well shielded from an explicit rationing of budgetary resources, which indicates that health care as social right is resilient to change. Such resilience has positive as well as negative consequences. It has guaranteed universal coverage for all citizens, but it has not allowed for flexibility in considering alternative models of care.

Resistance to Privatization

Health care policy disjunction, the difference between rhetorical commitments and political action, is not likely to be addressed by the direct and transparent commodification of health care services in Canada. However, the possibility merits some attention because there exists potential for increased indirect commodification, and many Canadians fear what they consider to be signs of 'slippage' into a U.S.-style system.

The levying of user fees and the practice of extra-billing in the provinces over the past two decades have been met with heavy resistance by the federal government, even though the actual instances and effects of extra-billing were negligible.[44] This has helped to reassure Canadians that the federal government is on moral high ground and is willing to impose its vision of citizenship on the provinces and enforce it with financial penalties. The degree to which the federal government will be able to defend citizens' rights against pressures for relaxed national standards in health care in the current fiscal context is a matter of ongoing debate.

Recent figures from Health Canada indicate that 'public sector health expenditures represented 69.9% of total health expenditures in

1996; with the public share continuing its downward trend from 74.6% in 1991,' while 'private sector health expenditures represented an estimated 30.1% of total health expenditures in 1996.'[45] That Canada has now fallen below 70 per cent in its public contribution to health care is significant because it seems to present a dangerous 'slippery slope' to increased commodification of health services; increased private sector involvement in an area of such import is unacceptable to many Canadians. Very shortly after the Health Canada document was released, the Canadian Institute for Health Information (CIHI), a government-funded not-for-profit organization that works very closely with Health Canada, produced data that suggest that the 'slight' decline in public expenditures noticed in 1996 would be arrested in the following year.[46] The CIHI explained that the more optimistic projections that it has prepared are 'more up to date than Health Canada's.'[47] Seemingly, the CIHI attempted to perform a damage control function for Health Canada (by confirming the more positive forecast), which had revealed figures that were, evidently, alarming for many. However, despite the efforts of CIHI, the potential for creeping privatization in the much revered universal health system seems to have been confirmed.[48]

One only needs to look as far as the United States to confirm fears of private control of medicine. Regularly, citizens in that country find themselves without adequate (or any) health insurance coverage, have their premiums increased because of 'risks' (i.e., illness or disease), or are dropped from private insurance plans altogether. Aside from these equity issues, the United States continues to spend upwards from 13.5 per cent of the Gross Domestic Product (GDP) on health care, or approximately $4,500 per capita,[49] the highest of all member countries of the Organization for Economic Cooperation and Development (OECD). The predominance of Health Maintenance Organizations (HMOs) over the past three decades has contributed to the diminishment of medical authority in the United States to such an extent that physicians in some states are trying to organize labour unions to counterbalance corporate power. In addition, there have been several attempts (at both federal and state levels) to adopt some aspects of the Canadian system in a movement towards universality. Such evidence seems to confirm the superiority of Canadian health care. However, there is no clear consensus on the importance of health care as a symbol of national identity in Canada. It might even be the case that Canadians are ready to accept a two-tiered system. In 1998 a study conducted by the Harvard School of Public Health found that 23 per cent of Canadians believed that the health care system needed to be completely rebuilt, 37 per cent thought that fundamental changes were needed, and 46 per cent stated that recent reforms diminished the quality of care.[50]

However, as Naylor states regarding public opinion polling, 'much depends on the wording.'[51] In a 1996 Gallup Poll, almost 60 per cent of Canadians rejected the concept of 'two levels of health care service: a basic one that government funded for everyone, and another under which those who could afford it paid the full amount and received whatever kind of services they wanted.'[52] In that same year, another Gallup Poll found that '44 percent of respondents favored a two-tier system (described as government insuring basic services, with private insurance or direct payment options available for further coverage). With this formulation, even supporters of the nominally socialist New Democratic party registered a 42 percent level of support for a two-tier plan.'[53]

Thus, what is of real importance is the rhetorical force of political arguments. From this study it can be concluded that citizens seem to want governments to remain committed to equity, but do not necessarily demand that every aspect of service provision be strictly equal. The numbers might not reflect levels of support for future directions for health care so much as they reflect support for the existing system, wherein everyone has the same basic coverage, with private insurance available for eyeglasses, eye examinations, dental services, chiropractic medicine, and the like.

The Politics of Retrenchment

The fiscal crisis, and hence political crisis, of the welfare state has been well documented.[54] In Canada, in the 1980s and the early to mid-1990s, unmanageable deficits and debt, lack of economic growth, and high rates of unemployment forced many governments to commit themselves to exercising fiscal restraint and pursuing policies of retrenchment. This meant significant reductions in funding for health care at both the federal and provincial levels at a time when medical technology was advancing rapidly and the population was aging (of course, technology for health care continues to advance, and the population continues to age). However, it is unlikely that with the recommitment of federal funding for health care the 'crisis' of the universal health system is over. In fact, governments that have successfully balanced their budgets and injected surpluses into the health care system have already demonstrated that demands on the health care system outpace governments' ability to provide funding. The clocks cannot be turned back for defenders of social rights.

The Political Implications of Federalism: Social Policy Stasis

The fiscal 'crisis' as it pertains to health care can be gleaned through the study of federal–provincial fiscal relations. Federal contributions to provincial health programs were established, at the outset (1966), on a cost-sharing basis, whereby the federal government matched provincial spending in the health field, and provinces were required to comply with national standards. The arrangements for public medical insurance established that the federal government would pay 50 per cent 'of the national per capita cost of insured services, multiplied by the insured population of the province,'[55] and the provinces were required to operate and manage their health care systems in accordance with program conditions.

With the implementation of Established Programs Financing (EPF) in 1977, the federal government was able to assume a greater degree of control over its spending on health care (under the former cost-sharing arrangements the provinces held the balance of power). The new fiscal arrangements resulted in the end of cost-matching for health care, and replaced the conditional scheme with a block-funding arrangement. There were three components to the EPF arrangements: a block grant, a tax point transfer, and an equalization component.

Block-funding arrangements are essentially unconditional in nature, which meant that with EPF the provinces were granted a significant degree of autonomy. However, the degree to which this was actually the case is a matter of perception. Some provinces considered the new fiscal arrangements for the established programs to be a victory: there was no longer any requirement that the funds be spent on the designated programs, and there was no penalty indicated for permitting user charges and facility fees.[56] However, other provinces were suspicious of the arrangements and believed that the federal contribution would not be sufficient to cover escalating costs.

Although the federal government's use of its spending power to direct provincial action has generated great controversy, much of the intergovernmental tension in the field of health care is the result of normative and symbolic disputes. For example, one of the most contentious 'illusions' of federal–provincial relations is the transfer of tax points provided for in the EPF arrangements. The federal government underestimated the yield of the tax points (13.5 per cent personal income tax and 1 per cent corporate income tax), which meant that the cash component remained a substantial portion of the total contribution much longer than expected. However, the cash component secured federal visibility in this important policy field, which was politically desirable for the federal government.

To most Canadians it appeared that in intergovernmental conflict regarding health care the federal government was concerned with moral standards while the provinces were concerned only about the funding arrangements. This, however, is not quite the case.

Thomas Courchene explains that the tax transfer is 'notional' in that 'the provinces are assumed to have taken up this vacated federal tax room.'[57] The revenue yielded by those tax points is provincial revenue, and not a federal contribution, although the federal government indicates otherwise. In the first year of the EPF arrangements the tax point transfer constituted a federal contribution of funds. But, after the initial transfer, the tax room created is properly considered to be within the provincial realm of taxing prerogatives. In federal calculations of EPF and CHST transfers, the tax points are included as part of the yearly transfer of funds for social programs. Hence, it appears in federal accounts that the federal government is transferring much more revenue to the provinces for health care services than is actually the case. This practice is what Stefan Dupré considers to be 'at the top of my list of the Big Lies of Canadian public finance.'[59]

In 1982 the federal government began applying the EPF escalator to the entire transfer, which caused the cash component to decline steadily. This also meant that federal visibility and program conditionality were declining. Because the transfer of tax points is inherently unconditional (it cannot easily be withheld), the federal government devised a new set of financial arrangements to secure the conditional cash portion. It is symbolically important that the federal government maintain the perception that national standards are being upheld. Miriam Smith explains the implications of the declining cash component of EPF: 'As the federal cash funding declines as a proportion of total federal expenditure, the federal government's ability to enforce the conditions of the Canada Health Act also declines.'[59] Or, in the words of Courchene, 'Ottawa's version of the "golden rule" is becoming less and less sustainable: as it stops supplying the gold, it is also losing its moral authority to make the rules.'[60]

The federal government addressed these problems with the fiscal arrangements in the 1995 budget. The CHST (implemented the following year) collapsed funding for health care, post-secondary education, and social assistance into a single transfer. This allowed the federal government to increase and maintain the cash component, which was expected to run out in 2010 under the EPF arrangements, while reducing the overall amount of the transfer.[61] The CHST does not make any distinctions among the three areas – provinces are free (read obligated) to set priorities and allocate funds as they deem appropriate. Under the new arrangements, it seems that health care has fared, and is likely to continue to fare, the best of all three programs.

Health care is Canada's success story. The country's record in the field of income maintenance, by way of comparison, is very poor. Income maintenance accounts for relatively low levels of social spending: 'It is Canada's relatively niggardly approach to income maintenance (other than unemployment insurance, or UI) that accounts for relatively low social spending levels.'[62] Canada's low level of social spending (relative to other OECD countries) is not the result of low levels in all three areas, but generous levels of health care spending and extremely low levels of spending on income maintenance programs.[63]

The implications of these 'two worlds' of social policy will likely appear in future restructuring agendas. For example, the population health model, which is an integrated framework that focuses on the determinants of health (socioeconomic status, and education, for instance)[64] was adopted by all Canadian governments in 1994.[65] Like the CHST, the population health framework amalgamates, in theory, all major social programs so that important connections can be made among them. However, in spite of explicit recognition of the importance of income maintenance spending and policy development in relation to health, it seems that governments have not channelled sufficient resources into these areas. Looking ahead, it is not likely that the priorities of social policy will change. Health care will remain the cornerstone of Canadian citizenship, and therefore command the attention of governments, while income maintenance/welfare assistance programs will further diminish as priorities.

Conclusion

The increases in federal cash commitments through the CHST (provided in the 1999 and 2000 federal budgets, and in the agreement reached at the September 2000 First Ministers Meeting) appear to have called an end to cutbacks in health care. With the infusion of additional cash payments, the federal government has renewed its commitment to social equity and universality. In addition, the agreement reached at the First Ministers Meeting in September 2000, in which the federal government allocated additional funding for health care, and the provinces agreed to prepare health care report cards (to improve accountability of provincial governments to their citizens, not to the federal government),[66] indicates that there is still political consensus that health care ought to be a priority, and thereby delivered as a public good, a social right of citizenship.

That consensus looks a lot like the status quo, although there is ongoing intergovernmental negotiation regarding the balance of federal and provincial authority for health care. For politicians, re-establishing or saving a revered social program from feared or disruptive changes will almost always be a sound move to garner public support. In Nova Scotia, for example, the current Progressive Conservative government campaigned on a platform that included commitment to undo major changes made to the health care system in the past 10 years; at the time of writing, the initial regionalization scheme was in the process of being dismantled. This tendency, to promise reversing unpopular reform, even if much needed, and then to be compelled to deliver on it, coupled with social rights defences, creates even greater policy stasis.

The strength and stability of the medical profession as a virtually unrivalled interest group in the health policy field is another major factor contributing to lack of much-needed change. In Chapter 6, the relationship between organized medicine and the state will be examined against epidemiological trends and public policy commitments to 'population health' and greater flexibility in service delivery. At an increasing rate, professional ethics are running headlong into governments' precarious funding arrangements and public health evidence that apparently prioritizes community health initiatives over individual needs. Thus, Chapter 6 introduces bioethical and interest group challenges for federalism.

6

Medicine, Health, and Inequality

Stasis, caused in part by social rights claiming, is problematic because it reinforces medical and institutional models of health care. This presents a paradox because at the same time that defenders of the social rights thesis criticize medical and institutional models, their defences of the right to health care actually serve to maintain those models. As explained in Chapter 2, citizens' expectations are rising; citizens expect that the health care system will keep pace with their demands and provide the latest medical technology, access to pharmaceuticals, and alternative medicines and services. At first glance, these expectations seem to be inconsistent with the medical model because they identify patterns of entitlement outside of the existing terrain (the current model of provision does not make universally available pharmaceuticals, alternative medications, and services provided outside of usual institutional settings). It would seem to be the case that citizens' expectations repudiate rather than perpetuate the medical model. However, citizens' expectations also remain constant over time. To take these points together, it is evident that citizens' expectations rise incrementally, meaning that expectations build on existing expectations rather than replace them. In addition, social rights claiming reinforces the medical model because the political importance of the right to health care is used or distorted by organized medicine to resist changes to its privileged position in the health care arena. For example, the Canadian Medical Association (CMA) can provide resistance to health care reform by claiming that reform efforts will compromise the ability of medical doctors to act in accordance with their professional ethics. Also, many physicians have an interest in maintaining the status quo because their incomes and careers depend on it.

The medical profession is a constraint in its own right. Its authority, conferred by its (scientific) expertise, historical pattern of dominance, and current status as single most important interest in the health policy field, accounts for stability in the system.[1] Clearly, it serves to maintain the medical model (which refers to care that is delivered by medical doctors in clinical settings, as well as the system of training, hierarchy, autonomy, and dominance that privileges medical doctors over other practitioners).[2] This is not to say that the medical profession is somehow malevolent, but that it has gained for itself a position of dominance in health care vis-à-vis other practitioner groups, and that this dominance has provided the health care system in Canada with a certain 'logic.'[3]

My argument is that assertions of health care rights by Canadians support rather than challenge the medical model. When citizens claim, in response to reform efforts, that they have the right to health care, they are expressing their discontent with the proposals, and their preference for the existing arrangements. There is further evidence that citizens have come to trust their physicians, and distrust their governments' abilities to deal with system reform. A recent opinion poll revealed that 'almost 80% of respondents were very or somewhat satisfied with the ability of the health care system to meet their or their family's needs. But only 62% were satisfied with the system's ability to meet the needs of all residents of the province.'[4] Similarly, another poll conducted in Ontario found that 81 per cent of respondents 'were satisfied with the outcome of their hospital stay ... [and] gave high ratings to the care they received from doctors and nurses.'[5]

Physicians are often identified as the 'gatekeepers' to the Canadian health care system. Patients must consult a general practitioner (GP) as their primary caregiver to gain access to specialists. This system ensures that GPs are the primary point of contact for patients in the system, regardless of the increasing popularity of other practitioners as primary caregivers (obstetricians and gynaecologists for women, nurse practitioners, chiropractors, physiotherapists, and nutritionists). In many cases, however, patients can opt for other caregivers, such as chiropractors and physiotherapists, without being referred through their GP, but they are not covered for those 'alternative' services under the public insurance plan.

This pattern of consultation and referral is definitive of the medical model for three reasons. First, it perpetuates the authority of medical doctors. Consequently, it is difficult for alternative patterns to be established. Nurse practitioners, nutritionists, and chiropractors, for instance, remain subordinate to medical authority because the care that they provide is either supplementary to, or effectively outside of, the existing structure of primary care. Second, the medical profession tends not to be focused on preventive care. Although there might be a culture change beginning as GPs demonstrate greater willingness to advise patients on nutrition, exercise, and alternative medications, physicians are trained to diagnose and treat disease, not prevent it.[6] In short, medical doctors are trained to focus on managing disease and illness (with surgery and pharmaceuticals) rather than managing patients. Third, such trends reinforce institutional patterns of care. Hospital and clinical settings are deemed most appropriate for treatment or cure.

The GP gatekeeping function is not without its benefits. Such a mechanism provides for good coordination of care, and it is cost effective because control can be exercised at the initial point of access. Consequently, it would not be wise to eliminate altogether the GP gatekeeping function. Rather, it might be necessary to examine possibilities for complementary avenues for alternative service provision and physician remuneration, given that there is greater need for other types of health care provision (while physicians and hospitals consume the vast amount of resources).

Expenditures for hospitals and physicians' services account for approximately 75 per cent,[7] of total provincial health budgets, clearly, the vast majority of health care resources. When governments make adjustments in these areas, physicians respond by recategorizing services and reallocating their time to maintain desired income levels. The autonomy of the profession, in addition to the fee-for-service method of payment, seems to make containment of supply practically impossible. In simple terms, the problem is that the incentive structure allows physicians to control levels of consumption of health resources, which means that momentum for change in the system builds towards expansion of medical services delivered in clinical settings and away from more integrative or collaborative approaches to health care.

The increase in rates of service growth, believed to be the result of raised citizens' expectations, positive political feedback for expanding health programs, changing demographics, and availability of new medical technologies, is largely the result of the way in which physicians are remunerated. Until pressures for growth of supply-side costs are removed, fundamental change will not likely be achieved. The remarkable stability of physicians' and institutional care costs (as proportion of expenditures), combined with difficulty in establishing incentives for physicians to practise in rural locations, and the renegotiation of collective agreements for health care workers according to equity criteria, leaves provincial governments tinkering with health care reform on the budgetary margins.

Medical Dominance and Democracy

The dominance of the medical profession and the perpetuation of the medical model raise questions concerning effectiveness and democracy. If expenditures for hospital and physicians' services consume vast proportions of health care budgets, then it seems that cost effectiveness and cost containment will be contingent on governments' ability to limit and reduce the supply of those services. If democratic values are being promoted within the health care system (as in the case of community governance structures – see Chapter 7), then the dominance of an elite group of decision-makers with no direct accountability to voters should be considered a problem.

As noted, the institutional dominance of physicians as the gatekeepers to the system has many advantages. It helps to control costs in that it maintains stable and predictable patterns of health services consumption. It establishes access to a range of caregivers through a medically trained generalist. Thus, the dominance of the medical profession can be justified by both fiscal imperatives and science. If such justifications are sound, then how can they be challenged?

In the case of the former (fiscal imperatives), it is not necessarily the case that the budgetary consistency afforded by the medical model precludes other cost-effective options. There might be several alternative configurations that would produce favourable results. Of course, there would be transition costs involved in redirecting resources from physicians and clinical settings to home care programs, for example. But as the needs of the population become more dynamic, it becomes evident that the medical model will require adjustment if the five principles of the Canada Health Act are going to continue to be upheld. Otherwise, the creation of new programs like home care and pharmacare that are outside of the purview of the act will expand private sector involvement in health care, and thereby raise questions about access and equity (although expenditures for hospitals and physicians will remain stable).

The second justification, that physicians have more scientific and medical training than other practitioners, and that this qualifies them to serve as trustees for the health care system, is also questionable. It makes sense to seek consultation for medical problems from appropriately trained medical personnel (it might not be wise for one to consult a nutritionist or a massage therapist to inquire about chest pains). However, the authority of medical doctors has not always been (and is not always) conferred by science. As Pat and Hugh Armstrong explain:

> Indeed, allopathic doctors' authority did not begin with their knowledge of scientific evidence. Rather, it preceded the development of the kinds of techniques on which today's medicine is based ... [For example] in 1865, organized medical men in Ontario were successful in getting the state to grant the exclusive right to attend childbirths. Because there was a surplus of graduates from medical school, they wanted not only to eliminate competition from the unorganized women who served as midwives but also to use childbirth as a way of becoming family practitioners. But this monopoly was not based on evidence that these allopathic practitioners were safer and more effective in attending birth. In fact, a Saskatchewan medical officer reported in 1919 that 'maternal mortality was much higher in the 50 per cent of confinements attended by medical men.'[8]

In the context of late twentieth/twenty-first century medicine, the scientific foundation of medicine has been established, but remains fallible. In the estimation of Armstrong and Armstrong, the foundation is not sound enough to justify the unchallenged dominance of the medical profession:

> Although there is clear evidence that many of the treatments provided by doctors are safe and effective today, it cannot be assumed that this is the case for all treatment. A report prepared recently for federal, provincial, and territorial deputy ministers of health concluded that, among doctors, there 'is a poor awareness of evidence about effectiveness, and there are few good mechanisms to implement changes in practice patterns among practising physicians.' In addition, it found a 'lack of uniform standards of clinical competence for licensure,' 'inadequate attention to self-regulation of practice to overlapping "scopes of capability" and the need for

continuing competence review,' and 'deficiencies in both the amount and quality of basic clinical and management information.' In other words, self-government was not ensuring quality. The gatekeepers to practice were not adequately keeping the gates.[9]

These problems with doctors' authority and expertise, in addition to the unsoundness of the scientific foundations of medicine, do not necessarily add up to a legitimacy crisis. To be sure, the practice and science of medicine cannot be expected to be perfect. To point out its flaws is not to dismiss the benefits that it provides. However, the problems mentioned do seem to indicate that a discussion needs to proceed about the desirability of continued dominance of the profession and about alternative medicine and configurations of service delivery. As Patricia O'Reilly points out, 'it needs to be kept in mind, both for historical record and for the understanding of today's health care issues, that unproven ideas are not necessarily erroneous ideas. Questions never asked are questions never answered.'[10]

One such alternative is the creation of community governance structures (discussed at length in the following chapter). By decentralizing service provision and decision-making authority, the state seems to be 'democratizing' certain elements of the health care system. This approach to structural reform will serve to challenge the medical model: decision-making will be more transparent and citizens will be able to contribute to discussions about health resources allocation in their communities, which might provide some balance or resistance to established patterns of medical dominance. However, that dominance might serve another purpose. Similar experiences in the United States in the 1960s and 1970s provide a warning. James Morone explains that with increased community engagement 'the medical profession lost its trusteeship over American medicine. In every community, groups of lay people were making judgments on proposals submitted by the medical professionals. In so doing, they were transforming the way Americans think about health care policy.'[11]

The result of the transformation was increased private control of medicine. Managed care corporations were able to assume the authority lost by organized medicine. The possibility that this will occur in Canada is worth considering. It is also appropriate to question whether it might be more difficult for governments to politically manage decision-making bodies by lay participants than to accommodate the interests of organized medicine.

Organized Medicine and the State

It might be that the medical profession has consolidated its authority to such an extent that governments have few options for major structural reform. However, the 1986 doctors' strike in Ontario is an example of conflict between the medical profession and the government, where organized physicians failed to win substantial concessions from the state.[12] This anomalous result is explained, in large part, by the factiousness of the medical profession.

At first glance, the profession seems to be a monolith of consolidated power, with which unwitting governments must bargain. However, on closer inspection it becomes clear that the medical profession is divided into various factions, each competing for policy concessions. According to Carolyn Hughes Tuohy, there are at least two distinct groups within the realm of organized medicine: the entrepreneurial majority, whose view 'is expressed a fortiori by the voluntary provincial medical associations,' committed to defending entrepreneurial discretion ('defending the institutions of private fee-for-service practice which allow the volume and mix of service to be used as instruments of income generation, although the price may be centrally negotiated');[13] and the 'strategic minority,' which is 'dedicated to the preservation of professional governance of the clinical discretion of physicians'[14] (usually, this minority consists of the regulatory colleges and the medical schools). The 'strategic minority' as the moral faction of the medical profession is regularly overshadowed by the 'entrepreneurial majority' in political debate. In fact, most of the tension between organized medicine and the state can be attributed to the confrontational entrepreneurial majority, as the more accommodating strategic minority has historically demonstrated 'a willingness to collaborate with governments, trading off some measure of the entrepreneurial discretion of individual physicians in order to maintain [clinical discretion].'[15]

The privileged position of medicine, which is not readily open to contest by other groups in the health sector,[16] has made supply constraints virtually unalterable by governments. Medical professions, as constituencies of federal and provincial levels of government, interact at a symbolic level and a practical level (bargaining is done at the provincial level by medical societies to determine fee schedules, for example). Historically, at the federal level national objectives are set to demonstrate symbolically consistent commitments. At the provincial level, governments are compelled to recognize these commitments in practice, according to the demands and preferences of citizens and organized interests in each province. This recitation of the original intergovernmental arrangements for health is a largely unpopular view among the provinces in the current context of reinterpreting the social union.[17]

Harvey Lazar has indicated that 'the federal government is torn between a more collaborative approach and its interpretation of a public mood which appears to want Ottawa to continue to play a 'strong' role to maintain one-tier health. What remains to be seen is whether it is possible for Ottawa to sustain a strong role while moving toward a more collaborative approach.'[18] It is not clear exactly what is envisioned with a 'more collaborative approach,' although the intergovernmental agreement reached in September 2000 seems to indicate that the federal government and the provinces are capable of accommodating one another (see Chapter 5). But it seems that when supply-side issues are taken into consideration, a diminished federal role would mean that the symbolic impact of a national vision for health care will be blunted, and physicians' opportunities to pursue self-interest (and to continue to propagate their pursuits) contrary to the social rights thesis, will increase. Fragmentation and lack of collaboration among provinces, which is not necessarily mitigated by the report cards, might enable more provider control.

At the level of provision, then, health care services are distributed or reallocated according to entrenched interests, on the one hand, and the changing expectations of citizens-as-patients, on the other. At this point there is a collision of the constraints established by government on the demand and supply sides of the health care equation. The availability of health care services, and the ways in which they are provided, directly affect the ways in which health care services are consumed. For example, the decision to limit the number of available acute care beds in each province is based on evidence that demand will expand to the capacity of supply: an empty hospital bed will always be filled. Patterns of utilization are determined by physicians (who recommend that their patients be admitted to hospital) as well as patients (who expect that they will have access to a full range of care).

However, as long as the current model of physician remuneration remains in place, viable alternatives will not be suggested by physicians, nor expected by patients. Physicians are educated according to the medical model of care, which is reinforced by the incentive structure for professional practice.[19] Moreover, the proportion of health care budgets that is allocated to hospital and physician services leaves little funding for alternatives such as community health centres or home care. Many provincial governments have reduced the number of available acute care hospital beds, yet they have not developed complementary or substitutive home care programs. Hence, patients and their families must assume greater responsibility for their care (following brief hospital stays, preparing for those stays, or in lieu of those stays) and the expense of that care, with insufficient resources and support.[20]

The lack of resources committed to home care programs has resulted in a new configuration of health care provision within the nursing profession. The serious underfunding of support services outside of hospital settings necessitates cheap labour sources, such as unregulated, poorly paid 'personal care workers' (PCWs) or 'unregulated care providers' (UCPs). As the traditional role of nurses changes to include nurse practitioners and PCWs, disruption and competition is created within the profession. Nurses with elevated status are being forced either to work at the lower end of the nursing hierarchy, or in nursing home and community settings, which alters the environment for service delivery. Janet Lum explains:

> In Ontario, there are two categories of licensed nurses: Registered Nurses (RNs) who have a minimum of three years of college or university training, and Registered Practical Nurses (RPNs, previously called nursing assistants) who take a 12- to 18-month college program. Data ... reveal [that] in 1992, there were 112,599 Registered Nurses (RNs) of whom 65% worked in hospitals, 6.9% in nursing homes and 10.1% in the community. By 1997, the total number of RNs in Ontario declined to 109,098, while the proportion of RNs working in hospitals decreased to 61.5%. At the same time, the percentage working in nursing homes increased (to 8.6%), as did the percentage of RNs working in the community (to 12.7%). These changes also affected employment status: in 1992, 55.7% of RNs working in Ontario indicated that they worked full-time while 31.5% worked part-time and 12.3% worked on a casual basis. By 1997, the proportion of full-time jobs had declined to 49.8% while the proportion of part-time jobs had increased to 33.3% and casual jobs to 14.2%.[21]

This pattern of change can also be observed among RPNs, which increases competition for jobs between RNs and RPNs. As hospitals deal with budget constraints, and search for the most efficient mix of hospital labour, nurses' unions try to defend the jobs of their members. This is a frustrating experience, which involves bargaining among nurses with different statuses within the profession. For example:

If hospitals must resort to UCPs as a cost-saving measure, the use of unskilled workers should be matched by the use of highly skilled RNs. In comparison to RPNs, registered nurses point out that they have greater breadth and depth of knowledge, can provide a wider range of care and are better trained to teach, delegate, assign and supervise UPCs. Supervision, they argue, is part of the basic entry level competency for RNs but not for RPNs. In response, RPNs maintain that many have taken additional professional development courses which include supervisory skills, and, that in their daily practice, they do supervise and provide other leadership skills of multi-disciplinary teams. RPNs make the additional claim that they are willing to do many of the 'lower level skills' which, in their view, RNs are increasingly unwilling to do – all at a more cost effective rate. In short, RPNs present themselves as a reasonable and safe compromise between more expensive RNs and low paid but untrained UCPs.[22]

On the one hand, the increased differentiation among nurses has had negative consequences generating competition among practitioners (often forced to level-down their qualifications) rather than uniting them in the face of such changes. Patricia O'Reilly identifies this as a

common pattern in twentieth century health care, that is, a hierarchically based gradation of clinical specialization within an already specialized segment of health care. As each subgroup within a group such as nursing moved up, another tended to move into the place it had vacated. As the rising status of the registered nurses, for example, left them reluctant to 'do the dirty work' of nursing, others came forth to perform the necessary tasks. So the assistants to the medical doctors began to require their own assistants. Even these assistants, the nurse's assistants, referred to today as practical nurses, now require the assistance of an orderly to whom they might assign unwanted tasks. All of this has set up a pattern of increased striation in health care.[23]

On the other hand, it has created more opportunities for nurses to advance their income and status according to skill levels (which now rival physicians). In 1992 the Ontario government passed legislation to support the role of nurse practitioners (NPs), which is an important step towards recognizing alternative methods of service provision in an overburdened health care system. NPs, now recognized in several provinces, 'are permitted to perform a broader range of services than registered nurses including the capacity to autonomously diagnose, treat, and prescribe medications for common illnesses in primary health care; and, under certain circumstances, order ultrasounds, x-rays, and laboratory tests.'[24] The introduction of nurse practitioners to the health system holds promise for addressing some perennial problems in the provision of Canadian health care services. The difficulty and expense of attracting physicians to rural locations is often addressed with NPs, as a cheaper alternative, and also as a more flexible alternative. Governments are committed on a rhetorical level to a more holistic approach to health care, which fits well with expanding alternatives for provision. However, the resistance of physicians to a more dynamic interpretation of health care (as a matter of professional ethics, status, and income) has resulted in seemingly impenetrable supply constraints. It is quite easy to understand that if physicians are compensated on a fee-for-service basis, they will be unwilling to share service provision with other practitioners. It is not exactly clear why governments are consistently quiescent to physicians' demands.

In 1997, five years after NPs were formally recognized in the Ontario health sector, the cap on physicians' income (which was instated in 1991) was raised, and the medical profession was given, through legislation, 'an effective 'veto' over proposed reforms which could potentially allow nurses to take on many of the primary care functions now controlled by physicians, including changes in doctors' roles in the health care system, alternative models of service delivery and compensation for services.'[25] This was clearly a decision in favour of increasing the strength of the medical profession relative to other groups in the health sector and in relation to government. By securing medicine's privileged bargaining position, the state commits itself to future spending and priority setting according to terms set by the medical profession. But why does the state continue to accommodate the medical profession?

Malcolm Taylor, Michael Stevenson, and Paul Williams provide some insight into this conundrum. In their consideration of the provincial variations in the relationship between organized medicine and the state, they suggest, 'that they are as limited as they are may be as much a reflection of the lack of serious political imagination and determination on the part of provincial governments in support of Medicare as it is a reflection of the resilience and ideological opposition to Medicare of the medical profession.'[26] Further, the dominance of the medical profession is distinctly political in that it concerns the allocation (by government) of scarce resources and the criteria by which those resources are distributed. And in this way, consideration of the relationship between the medical profession and the government sheds light on the larger rationing issues that are pressing in the Canadian context. Budget balancing and surplus management are the preoccupations of governments, and health sectors are particularly volatile in this budgeting environment, given the fiscal resources that they consume. This situation, juxtaposed to the popularity of health care programs, explains why rationing is done at the margins of budgets and on the demand side of the equation.

The Resilient Medical Model

Inauguration into the medical profession involves physicians making pledges of non-malfeasance and beneficence to their profession. The Hippocratic oath, often translated as the promise to 'first, do no harm,' and the commitment to beneficence (kindness, goodness, compassion) apply on a case-by-case basis. These commitments are understood to be deontological rather than consequential;[27] each patient is treated as an end in herself or himself, and not as a means to achieving a larger goal, such as that of population health. Trust in the medical profession is contingent on physicians' freedom to act in accordance with these categorical imperatives.

It is not surprising, then, that when governments begin to alter or reform the ways in which health care services are provided, physicians delegitimize the process by claiming that the proposed changes threaten to seriously restrict their ability to act in accordance with their professional commitments impoverishing the quality of service they provide. As a matter of strategy, physicians label government encroachments on their financial autonomy as threats to professional ethics. Such defences by physicians and their medical associations of the freedom to determine fee schedules, location of practice, and income levels, serve to undermine public confidence in government reform initiatives. They also serve to further strengthen the position of the medical profession and, consequently, citizens' defences of their rights to health care.

The Population Health Model

In 1994, all of the provinces agreed, in principle, to structure their health care reform agenda according to the population health model. The health promotion model, which predated the development of the population health model, requires that citizens take responsibility for their health and the health of their communities, which makes necessary some mechanism for assessing community needs and determinants of health. This means that, on the one hand, citizens must choose to adopt healthier lifestyles so that their need for medical care is reduced and, on the other hand, because resources are scarce and rationing involves distributing health services according to values, citizens and communities must be consulted in order to determine which values will direct the process.

Michael Hayes and Sholom Glouberman explain that 'while health promotion recognized that there were many determinants of health, it did not engage in the empirical research necessary to identify and explain the correlation between levels of socioeconomic status and measures of health status. Population health amasses population-based evidence in a systematic way in an attempt to identify and explain inequalities in health.'[28] Governments adopted in the 1990s the population health model,   to the dismay of many physicians caring for individual patients. As already pointed out, the population health approach promotes a broadened focus: social determinants of health, such as socioeconomic status, are considered to be of foremost importance within this framework. The problem, as identified by T.L. Guidotti, a physician, is that 'the model provided for the relationship between social and individual factors in health does not distinguish between the individual and the "population," and thus confuses individual "health and function" with population health status.'[29] For doctors, who see individual patients (with various conditions) on a daily basis, the population health model is an abstraction that fails to recognize the roles and experiences of front-line service providers.

In addition, and perhaps more troubling, there is a serious imbalance between federal spending commitments for social programs and

the provincial policy agenda. The policy directives of the social determinants of health framework necessitate strengthened financial and
moral commitments to social welfare and income maintenance programs. This clearly has not been achieved with the Canada Health and
Social Transfer (CHST), the funding arrangement that seemingly
broadened the social policy focus in the country but in reality, has significantly reduced the total amount of the transfer and forced difficult
allocation decisions onto provincial governments (as explained in
Chapter 5, provinces must now set priorities among three areas rather
than two).

The CHST was implemented at the same time that there was a public
policy paradigm shift in the field of health care. The amalgamated
transfer collapsed funding for health, post-secondary education, and
social assistance and, not coincidentally, the population health framework, which recognizes socioeconomic status and level of education as
determinants of health, was adopted by all Canadian governments.[30]
The population health approach (also referred to here as the determinants of health approach) differs from the traditional medical model in
at least two ways:

1 Population health strategies address the entire range of factors
   that determine health. Traditional health care focuses on risks and
   clinical factors related to particular diseases.
2 Population health strategies are designed to affect the entire population. Health care deals with individuals one at a time, usually individuals who already have a health problem or are at significant risk
   of developing one.[31]

The single most important determinant of health, according to the
framework document, is income and social status. People of low socioeconomic status (SES) have poorer health than those who are further
up the social and income hierarchy. At one time it was believed that
this difference in health was attributable to higher rates of smoking
and alcohol consumption, poor diet, and higher levels of stress in the
lower strata of the population.[32] However, research shows that when
these factors are controlled in both high and low SES populations, the
result is that people in the lower SES groupings still have poorer
health.

The data suggest 'some underlying general causal process, correlated with hierarchy, which *expresses* itself through different diseases.

But the particular diseases that carry people off may then simply be alternative pathways or mechanisms rather than 'causes' of illness and death; the essential factor is something else.'[33] And it is this 'something else' on which current public policy agenda should be focused.

Thus, public policy has been rhetorically reoriented to target certain disadvantaged populations, such as Native Canadians and children, so that the entire Canadian population will become healthier. Essential to this program is recognition of the differences among various ethnic, cultural, and socioeconomic populations, as well as important linkages between several policy areas: health, education, labour, income assistance, environment, and the economy. The population health strategy cannot be pursued solely within health portfolios; virtually all departments of the state must engage to achieve population health goals.

This integrated approach also includes increased emphasis on health promotion for all citizens. If people exercise more, eat a low-fat diet, smoke less, and learn to cope effectively with stress, then the overall demand for medical treatment will diminish. But, clearly, the research suggests that the first component of the strategy (recognizing socioeconomic determinants) is the more important. If levels of status and income are correlated with health, then governments should be committed to eradicating poverty and increasing the standard of living for all Canadians. However, Canada's record for income maintenance spending and program development for recipients of welfare is quite dismal, and it is not likely to improve under the current funding arrangements. Therefore, although federal and provincial governments remain committed to the rhetoric of the population health model, the extent to which governments are committed to implementing an integrated approach to social policy-making and service provision is not clear.

What would this approach mean for social rights? On the one hand, it reasserts the profundity of social class, and on the other, it verifies the need for public policy to address and incorporate other sources of inequality. The constraining effect of federalism, observable in the reduction in federal funding for health care at the same time that the population health model is being endorsed, makes the approach difficult to implement. The gap between rhetoric (of both social rights claims and reform) and action seems to be widening.

What is needed, then, is an approach that serves not to dismantle the medical model, but to recognize and institutionalize health promotion strategies. However, this broad, population-based approach needs to constitute only one element of a health policy reorientation. Guidotti's concerns about subordinating individual patients and their care to population health (a series of health indicators that amalgamate and dissolve the experiences of individuals and their particular relationships with physicians), are substantial. Therefore, there must be attempts, through public policy, to achieve balance. To continue with the AIDS example (the most notable exception to the trend from communicable to non-communicable disease), it is clear that health promotion strategies are crucial (i.e. public health campaigns advocating safe sex, clean needles), and need to target certain segments of the population. But public health needs must be balanced with individual concerns, like privacy, treatment, and choice.

Health Indicators and the Changing Contours of Disease

This lack of clarity of objectives and political capacity for implementation pose significant problems. A population health approach, with careful focus on social determinants of health, is likely what is needed in Canada, given the dynamics of the epidemiological transition. The World Health Organization (WHO) finds that, 'non-communicable diseases are expected to account for an increasing share of the disease burden, rising from 43% in 1998 to 73% by 2020, assuming a continuation of recent downward trends in overall mortality.'[34] This shift in main causes of death from communicable to non-communicable diseases has consequences for health, equity, and entitlement. According to the WHO document:

> The steep projected increase in the burden of noncommunicable diseases worldwide – the epidemiological transition – is largely driven by population ageing, augmented by the rapidly increasing numbers of people who are at present exposed to tobacco and other risk factors, such as obesity, physical inactivity and heavy alcohol consumption ... Health systems must adjust to deal effectively and efficiently with the globally changing nature of illness, and health policy-makers will be challenged to find the most cost-effective uses of their limited resources to control the rising epidemics of noncommunicable diseases.
>
> At the same time, health policy-makers will need to respond to the unexpectedly persistent inequalities in health status *within* countries ...

Recent studies have revealed surprisingly large inequalities within developed nations, and they highlight the need for policies that focus on disadvantaged populations throughout the world.[35]

Health

Two clear directives can be gleaned from this transition. First, individuals must take greater responsibility for their health by eating well, exercising more, reducing consumption of tobacco and alcohol, and taking precautions to reduce the spread of communicable diseases, such as HIV/AIDS. Second, governments must, through redistributive measures, provide resistance to the increasing polarization of the wealthy and the poor in society, so that overall health will improve, thus addressing non-communicable disease. This would also necessitate health promotion campaigns and programs that will fill the widening gaps in entitlement, such as well-developed home care and pharmacare programs. It seems to be the case that those with the most limited resources have the greatest difficulty obtaining home care services and appropriate pharmaceuticals.

Equity and Patterns of Entitlement

By addressing the social components of health, governments achieve equity, meaning fairness, rather than strict equality or sameness. Although attention still ought to be paid to reducing gaps in status and income, consonant with T.H. Marshall's analysis, social class should not be the sole lens through which inequality is examined in society.

Differences in income, health status, gender, race, sexuality, and ability, intersect and, as will be explained in Chapter 7, effectively create 'communities' that fall into marginal entitlement zones. Patients with AIDS, for example, need not only prohibitively expensive medication, but often need extensive home care services. Not all Canadians have access to a comprehensive range of health services, but they do have access to a limited range of medical and hospital-based services. The standard of expected service gets higher with improvements in medical technology which, paradoxically, make many medical and hospital-based services unnecessary.

It is likely that traditional patterns of health care service provision and utilization will continue to be replaced with a variety of new options, for which the state might be unwilling or unable to provide funding. The point is that this challenge cannot be addressed with what the WHO calls 'classical universalism.' Rather, 'new universalism,' which recognizes diversity and 'governments' limits but retains government responsibility for the leadership and finance of health systems,'[36] might replace Marshall's welfare state citizenship model.

These directives concerning health, and statements about equity and entitlement, are indications of a new blend of individual responsibility-taking (individual health and choice) and collective entitlement (health care distributed 'universally' as a public good). The right to health care, as an essential component of Canadian citizenship, manifests some aspects of this new blend, even if defenders of the right do not recognize the subtleties or complexities of their own claims. The substance of these claims, however, needs to be clarified, so that governments can implement reforms that will improve health in accordance with the changing epidemiological contours of disease.

Health and Empowerment

Just how new is the concept of individual empowerment for health care? Was it really absent from 'passive' welfare state arrangements? It might be argued that there has always been caregiving work done by friends and family members (often the burden has fallen disproportionately on women). This is certainly true. Nevertheless, the argument presented in the next chapter concerning the development of a more active, duty-bound citizenry, bolsters the claim made in this chapter, namely, that citizens *are* becoming more active in providing care as a means of adjusting to shorter patient stays, day surgeries, and outpatient services with meagre support for home care. Of course, to say that citizens *ought to* be more active in decision-making regarding health care is much different from saying that citizens *are* taking more and more responsibility in acquiring services (either by providing services 'free' for family members or paying for them to be provided by other care workers). In the paragraphs that follow I will explain how these claims are very different, yet connected.

Citizens are taking more responsibility for their own health care and the health of family members for two reasons. First, reduction in services provided in hospitals means that many services will be provided in the home. This includes preparation for surgery and treatment for recovery. Second, evidence shows that lifestyle is a main determinant of health, therefore, it is necessary for individuals to try to improve the conditions that may make them prone to disease as defined by the epidemiological transition. Both of these reasons for increased individual responsibility-taking for health require coincident state action. In the first instance, the state needs to adequately support family caregivers through well-developed home care programs. The second reason necessitates action in the direction of reducing income disparity within society.[37]

In determining how to distribute resources in society, it is necessary to define the communities among which public goods will be allocated. As argued, the universal distribution of health care services is being challenged by rising expectations, cost-containment policies, and differentiated citizenship claims. Strictly equal health care benefits are neither consistently valued by Canadians,[38] nor affordable, nor desirable in the current stage of citizenship development.

This approach is important, and not only because it indicates that there needs to be some mechanism for identifying and consulting various communities so that policy outcomes will reflect 'difference.' Engaging communities in decision-making for health care is also potentially empowering and edifying for citizens. Participation enables people to affect health care policy and restructuring efforts, as well as identify with the goals of reform. Taken together, citizen engagement can lead out of stasis because empowerment and consultation can provide some balance to the power of the medical profession. However, the argument presented is not that citizen or community authority should replace that of organized medicine, but rather that more effective citizen or community influence upon the state could ensure that the state itself acts as a more effective counterbalance to organized medicine.

Conclusion

Ethical, epidemiological, and professional assessments of health care dilemmas rarely offer compatible solutions. With such great diversity and disagreement in the health care policy field, where can reformers begin to look for answers?

In the next chapter, I will examine the potential of citizen and community participation in regional health authorities as a means of fostering deliberation and paths to policy decisions. This examination will also serve to evaluate the implications of the stasis that has resulted from failure to revise Marshall's thesis. As explained, social rights stasis has perpetuated existing (traditional) patterns of medical authority and service provision. I will argue that one main component of provincial reform agendas, the creation of community governance structures within regionalized systems, provides additional evidence of the changing mix of individual responsibility-taking and collective entitlement, and it has the potential to change the essential quality of social citizenship with more active modes of health care decision-making.

7

Citizenship, Entitlement, Community: Evaluating Community Governance Structures

The social rights thesis, coincident with the development of the welfare state, was designed to protect a certain relationship between citizens and the state. In Canada, this relationship can be discerned in debates concerning the universal health care system. Two general comments can be made about this relationship. First, this relationship serves to ensure equality. Citizens have come to expect that government will maintain commitments to universality in health care, and governments continue to promise that they will do so. Second, the relationship is defined by passivity, reinforced by the executive system of government. Because it was the entitlement side of T.H. Marshall's citizenship equation that became institutionalized in Canada, the right to health care came to be identified with a virtually unlimited set of expectations, with no corresponding, well-developed, notion of duty. It might be the case that citizens have fulfilled obligations (have paid for health care through their taxes) and that it is the entitlement side that is thin.

In any case, paying taxes in return for social programs is a relatively passive exchange. Marshall's theorizing might have engendered such passivity, although it was originally intended in much different (post–Second World War) circumstances. Marshall also believed that citizenship was an evolving concept, but he did not speculate about the configuration of citizenship beyond the period of social rights development. How may citizenship be conceived at the beginning of the twenty-first century?

Provincial exercises in community engagement for health care decision-making might provide important opportunities for citizens to fulfil their duties of citizenship. Citizens can become more active in determining the ways in which health care is delivered in the context of technological advancement, provision of alternative services, changing demographic and epidemiological patterns, and finite resources. The problem is that such opportunities may be undermined by social rights expectations, which perpetuate the existing welfare state model.

In this chapter, I examine the creation of community governance structures in Nova Scotia and Saskatchewan against the Medicaid rationing process undertaken in Oregon, to determine the possibilities for such exercises in the Canadian context. I have chosen Nova Scotia and Saskatchewan as case studies because each is an example of a different model of citizen involvement. Nova Scotia illustrates the process of citizen *input*, and Saskatchewan represents structures that have been created for citizen *governance*.[1] The Oregon experiment is an important example of transparent and community-level rationing. It provides lessons for countries such as Canada that, because of complex political factors, are being forced to recognize that (1) priority setting for health care is a value-laden process that may necessitate citizen involvement; (2) shifting difficult decisions onto citizens and their communities (under the guise of democracy) lets governments deflect some political 'heat' in this volatile policy area: and (3) prospects for public debate are contingent on institutional and structural factors, and they may not always achieve desired effects.

In the Canadian case community participation has the potential to contribute to the construction of an active conception of citizenship. This would be a major departure from the passive conception that is endemic to existing welfare state programs. However, the degree to which the much-needed debate concerning the future of universal health care can produce viable or useful results in community governance structures, regardless of their conceptual compatibility or incompatibility with social rights, is unclear.

Social Rights Versus Participation

It would appear that social rights are in conflict with participation. Social rights require little in exchange for benefits. The very idea of social rights is that a range of social services should be granted to all citizens, on the same terms, and not contingent on need, wealth, or income. At first glance, this is at odds with participatory expressions of citizenship. In a context where participation is valued, and where participation either directly or indirectly affects the decisions that are made, the guarantee provided by social rights is overridden. However, as explained later in this chapter, perhaps social rights and participatory modes of citizenship can be complementary rather than contradictory.

Despite possibilities for the compatibility of 'competing' approaches, it is necessary to decide which conception of citizenship will guide health policy decisions. The social rights conception is implicit in many of the significant scholarly contributions in the field. For instance, the compelling work of Pat and Hugh Armstrong rests on the assumption that health care should continue to be distributed as a public good, a social right of citizenship. However, the Armstrongs clearly 'reject the notion of simple choices between such alternatives as prevention and cure; promotion and intervention,'[2] which might also logically extend to the social rights – participation dichotomy. In addition, the work of Miriam Smith (which focuses on health care as an issue of federalism) and Robert Evans (which focuses on the economic viability or rationality of universal health care), while not squarely addressing the question of entitlement, lend support to uncritical defences of the social rights thesis. In neglecting the question of the validity or benefit of the entrenched right to health care, these analyses, building on unexamined assumptions, contribute to further misinterpretation.

Those who are concerned with participation seem to be uninterested in the symbolic value of health care, social rights, or citizenship. While all of these scholars raise important questions concerning citizen engagement and regionalization strategies, none of them employs a framework that can directly address the larger questions or issues of entitlement. I will try to bridge this gap by considering both health care as a social right of citizenship and citizen participation in health care decision-making.

Changing Health Care Decision-Making Structures in Canada

Public health insurance is guaranteed to all Canadians as a social right of citizenship. Therefore, any attempts to redesign the health system can be perceived as violations of that right. Governments proceed with caution to avoid inflaming public sentiment; they want to be re-elected. Public health insurance is universally available, and the middle class (which constitutes the largest group of voters) benefits greatly from the program.[3] Health care in Canada is perceived to be a right, and it is clearly valued by a majority of citizens for the tangible benefits that it provides.[4] With this in mind, it is tempting to ask, Why rock the boat? Let us dismiss the idea of developing citizen fora and community participation as a political mechanism for expressing criticism and making difficult decisions, and thus we can avoid alienating the majority of voters. Surely it is not that simple. In many Canadian provinces regional and community health boards have been created. These boards are the result of citizen demands for inclusion and governmental commitments to more openness and transparency in health care decision-making. These boards provide people with unique opportunities to fulfil their duties of citizenship.

Most governments in Canada are committed to formally engaging communities in decision-making processes concerning issues of distributional equity, namely, in the area of health care policy. In part, this is consistent with international trends towards greater transparency and community involvement in the distribution of health care resources and the recognition that priority setting for health care services is a value-laden process. It is also part of a larger governmental strategy of managing cutbacks, whereby difficult decisions that involve the limiting or elimination of health care services will be seen to be made by citizens and their communities.

The rhetoric of this strategy mimics closely the pioneering reforms undertaken in Oregon (which will be considered in a subsequent section). The literature outlining plans for regionalization and reform in Nova Scotia, for example, makes frequent mention of the need to define core services and to involve citizens in decision-making processes. However, virtually every attempt to distinguish core from non-core services has failed to achieve intended results.[5] In the Oregon case, the decision to fund one item and not another is based solely on fiscal criteria, and is thus entirely arbitrary from either a moral or clinical point of view.[6] It is not clear what Canadian reformers hope to achieve. Both outcomes and opportunities for engagement are important. The focus should be on decision-making processes and on what can realistically be achieved through community engagement exercises.

To what degree the rationing experiment in Oregon has affected Canadian reform efforts is difficult to determine. It is, however, likely that reformers in Canada's western provinces, if not in others, were well informed about it. There is no tangible evidence of this; Canadian reformers did not simply import the Oregon model and map it onto their political landscape, nor did they refer explicitly to it as a point of reference. Nevertheless, the rhetoric that makes the creation of community governance structures in Canada buoyant is remarkably similar to that used in the Oregon process – in contradistinction to that of European health care reform, for example.

The U.S. penetration of Canadian political discourse is a historical commonplace, and the prevailing view is that Canada–U.S. economic and political influences and relations are increasing in strength.[7] The market-driven approach to health care has long been the signature of the U.S. health care system, and now we see it in the creation of private clinics in Canada where physicians work in the for-profit health care business. In addition, the large migration of Canadian health care practitioners to the United States continues.

Engaging the Community: The Case of Nova Scotia

In the late 1980s and early 1990s, provincial governments were beginning to come to terms with health care as a fiscal issue in its own right, rather than as the by-product of intergovernmental discord. The federal government had been consistently reducing transfer payments to the provinces for social programs since 1977. Initial adjustments in the fiscal arrangements were likely related more to the budgetary planning themes that were in vogue at the time than to any long-term understanding of the demographic and technological developments that would expand health care budgets beyond fiscal capacity.

The fiscal conservatism of the federal Progressive Conservative government (1984–1993) had profound effects in Nova Scotia, a province that is dependent on federal equalization payments and social policy transfers for economic stability. Reductions in federal transfer payments, in the context of turbulent and frequent changes in provincial government leadership, resulted in well-intentioned, but never fully implemented, health reform agendas.

Groundwork for health care reform was set in 1989 with the Report of the Nova Scotia Royal Commission on Health Care, which recommended that citizens be included and thereby empowered in decisions regarding health issues.[8] The commission envisioned an expanded information network so that citizens would have access to information on health status, health costs, and the like, which would compel them to take more responsibility for their health choices. This conception of citizen empowerment was to be mobilized with decentralization of decision-making and the creation of regional structures for service delivery. These recommendations were reiterated and elaborated in the 1994 report of the Blueprint Committee on Health System Reform. The creation of Nova Scotia's 'blueprint' was itself an open and inclusive process; the substance of the report was based on extensive community interaction. According to the report, 'nearly 200 written submissions were received from individuals, municipal governments, health planning groups and a wide range of care providers. The vast majority supported the reform process and offered valuable suggestions for improving the health system. Many submissions highlighted the need for communities and consumers to have access to, and control over, health care services.'[9]

The government's response to this public sentiment was to create community governance structures within the regionalized health care system. The mandate for the new institutional design included the following: 'to allow for effective community input into decision-making about health care resource allocation.'[10] More specifically, and prior to regionalization, the Blueprint Committee recommended that regional health boards (RHBs) be created to establish, in consultation with the Department of Health, a list of core services that will be provided and funded categorically in all regions: 'The government's health policy included a commitment to establish *core services*. These are defined as essential health care services that must be provided throughout the province at a consistent standard. The *Blueprint* recommended that the RHBs and the Department of Health work together to identify core services at the community, regional and provincial levels and to develop a mechanism for funding these services.'[11]

This ambitious mandate would be supported by several community health boards (CHBs) in each region. According to the Blueprint Committee these would be responsible for:

> planning, coordinating, and authorizing the funding for primary health care in their area. To do this, an allocation for primary health care will be developed for each CHB by the RHB. Some examples of primary health care include outpatient clinics, physiotherapy services, nutrition programs, and well-baby clinics. Local primary health care providers, such as community health centres, will work with their local CHB by identifying the programs and services they can deliver most efficiently, effectively, and affordably.[12]

Clearly, in Nova Scotia the original mandate of RHBs and CHBs was to set priorities among health care spending areas. The rhetoric indicates that citizens and their communities, via these new community governance structures, would be the source of any new allocative decisions for health care services, if not the primary decision-makers in priority-setting exercises, with the Department of Health in a formal supervisory role. Daily political debate includes discussion of community involvement in setting priorities for health, and publications from the Department of Health regarding the reforms are littered with references to grassroots decision-making and community empowerment, which indicates a strong political commitment to engaging communities in difficult decision-making processes. This engagement can also be considered to be an attempt by the state to deflect or download difficult decision-making responsibilities onto those who are least equipped to make them. However, at this stage in the reform process there is need for neither praise nor alarm.

In Nova Scotia the implementation process began in 1996. At that time four RHBs were created, which were intended to organize all the province's health care facilities and resources into four distinct regional entities, each reporting to the province on behalf of hospitals and clinics.[13] This meant four bodies reporting to, and making demands on, the Department of Health rather than the thirty-six individual hospital boards that effectively performed these functions prior to regionalization.

However, at approximately the same time that the Department of Health was regionalized, several hospitals merged into larger regional entities and replaced a number of smaller institutions.[14] These new regional hospitals,[15] in addition to two other major hospitals in Halifax,[16] did not want to channel their efforts through the new health boards – there are obvious advantages in having *direct* access to government. Therefore, the province's four major health care complexes chose to remain outside the regional structure, effectively undermining the province's restructuring effort, and depriving the regional and community health boards of institutional support. The defiance of these four hospitals or non-designated organizations (NDOs) frustrated the Department of Health's entire reform agenda. NDOs directed and consumed a significant portion of the health care budget, yet remained outside the regional configuration.

The latest reorganization, which began 21 October, 1999, created nine District Health Authorities (DHAs). The new organizational structure consists of nine districts that fall roughly along established county lines. Government explicitly recognizes that the Department of Health holds ultimate authority and responsibility for all decisions concerning distribution.[17] Perhaps what is most significant is that the NDOs will be brought into the new system, so that they will work with and not against the DHAs. Unfortunately, the latest reform efforts constitute yet another major disruption in the health care system.

The Case of Saskatchewan

Saskatchewan, distinguished as the birthplace of public health insurance in Canada, consistently draws attention in the social policy arena. The province's cooperative political culture, resource-based economy (vulnerable to boom-and-bust cycles), and commitment to social progress, make it exceptional from other provinces.

In 1995 Saskatchewan became the first province to balance its budget, and it remains the only province to have done so before beginning systematic health care reform. Moreover, the New Democratic Party government eliminated the budget deficit while it remained dedicated to social democracy in a politically, socially, and economically conservative context.

The most significant differences between community engagement in health care decision-making in Nova Scotia and Saskatchewan are briefly explained in the paragraphs that follow. First, in Saskatchewan, legislation compelled all providers to operate within the regionalized structure, which prevented the undermining of the reform process that characterized the Nova Scotia experience. Second, budgeting decisions were devolved to the districts in Saskatchewan (there are thirty-two). Each district board includes some members appointed by the Department of Health (one-third) and some elected by the district constituency (two-thirds).[18] In Nova Scotia full decision-making authority for budgetary allocations rests with the Department of Health (this was reaffirmed with the October 1999 reorganization). Third, in Saskatchewan, there was clear agreement among decision-makers that deficit reduction was not health care reform; therefore, the provincial budget was balanced before health system reform was undertaken. The fourth important difference that accounts for Saskatchewan's success in regionalizing its health care system and encouraging citizen participation was the political stability in that province during the policy planning and implementation phases. The Roy Romanow NDP government enjoyed a firm hold on power from 1991 to 1999, during which time there were relatively few administrative rearrangements. In that same period in Nova Scotia there were four different governments, continuous reshuffling of cabinet and senior levels of the public service, and departmental reorganizations. According to one official who attended the meetings of health ministers, there was a completely different group (deputy minister and other senior officials) from Nova Scotia each year.[19]

The fifth and final difference is that the Saskatchewan government began with principles for reform, rather than a detailed blueprint. In Saskatchewan, those involved in policy planning realized that a detailed blueprint could not be implemented. This effectively prevented a situation wherein government becomes inflexible throughout the reform process because it committed at the outset to unachievable goals. Health care reform was properly realized as an evolutionary process through which compromises would have to be made in accordance with a consistent set of principles. Thus, implementation of district health boards in Saskatchewan has been a success relative to other provincial experiences. Furthermore, in Saskatchewan district health board members are elected, a stated goal of most other provincial regionalization plans.

There are, however, two major problems that have not yet been adequately addressed in this evaluation of regionalization health care services in Saskatchewan. The first involves the distribution of health care resources. In times of retrenchment, when there is no money to spend, allocation is rather simple: cuts are made to areas and agencies that will have the least negative political impact. When there is a budget surplus and a small amount of money to be spent, which is now the case, decision-making becomes soberingly difficult. The second problem is the potential power imbalance that will eventuate among communities, the state, and organized medicine. As experiences in the United States warn, replacing state dominance by community authority, while at the same time decreasing the influence of organized medicine, makes for a relatively unstable – and ultimately impotent – tripartite relationship.[20]

The Case of Medicaid Reform in Oregon: Rationing Resources

Medicaid is a joint federal–state program developed in the United States in the 1960s to assist disadvantaged groups such as the poor and the disabled. Guidelines for entitlement are set federally, but eligibility is determined by individual states. Consequently, there is enormous variation in eligibility requirements among states, although the range of services available to those who are eligible is comprehensive and consistent.

Prior to 1996, federal law required that all persons eligible for Aid to Families with Dependent Children (AFDC), blind or disabled persons with incomes below a level determined by the state, and women and children covered by the federal Poverty Level Medical Program (states cannot adjust the eligibility threshold for this program) were the intended recipients of Medicaid support.[21] The largest group of Medicaid recipients were AFDC-eligible persons, and each state was responsible for determining the eligibility threshold for its AFDC and hence Medicaid recipients. In 1995 the federal poverty level for a single adult was U.S. $6,620 per year; and for a family of four it was U.S. $12,000. That same year Oregon set its requirement for AFDC at 58 per cent of the federal poverty level; therefore, a family that made over U.S. $6,960 per year was ineligible for public funding.[22] In Alabama the income threshold for AFDC was set at 14 per cent of the federal poverty level.[23] To deal effectively with escalating health costs and heavy resistance of citizens to increased taxation in the 1980s, state governments had available few instruments to deal with the fiscal situation. Indeed, the Oregon Health Services Commission recognized at the outset of the reform process that 'society's expectations are on an inevitable collision course with its resources, and that something must be done.'[24]

The most common response by state legislatures to uncontrollably expanding expenditures was to further reduce the eligibility threshold for AFDC. 'Unfortunately this [was] often the easiest solution politically, and the effects can be extreme.'[25] The state of Oregon, led in its boldness by Senator Kitzhaber, decided that exercising fiscal restraint by penalizing the most disadvantaged persons in society was neither politically nor morally viable. Something different would have to be done.

In September 1988 the Oregon Medicaid Priority-Setting Project was established to consider and rank a variety of health care benefits for Medicaid recipients. In addition, the legislature 'established an 11-member Health Services Commission (HSC) whose goal was twofold: expand Medicaid coverage and establish a list of prioritized health care services, to be periodically reviewed.'[26] The basic premise on which this group was given its mandate was that the state should guarantee at least a basic set of publicly insured services to all citizens who cannot afford or are not eligible for private insurance or Medicaid.

At that time, only certain low-income groups were eligible for public funding under Medicaid, which consisted of a virtually unlimited range of health services. This left an estimated 400,000 Oregonians uninsured.[27] The state decided that the federal program should be restructured so that all individuals and families whose income was below the federal poverty line would be entitled to public insurance. The system was to be transformed from one that distributed benefits according to a person's eligibility to one that distributed or rationed services across a wider population.

From 1989 through 1993 the Oregon HSC worked at drafting a comprehensive and viable list of health services, ranked from most important to least important. The final list (approved in 1993) was considerably different from the first attempt which (as result of counterintuitive ranking) was dismissed outright.[28] Yet despite many fundamental changes in methodology and orientation throughout the process, the commitment to recognizing and incorporating community values in the priority-setting exercise remained constant. Citizen participation was indispensable partially by virtue of that state's political culture,[29] and partially it was a manifestation of the current international trend towards more transparency and openness in restructuring health care systems.

The forerunner to and impetus for the Oregon plan was Oregon Health Decisions (OHD), 'a network of citizens aiming to raise awareness of bioethical problems among the public.'[30] In 1987 OHD began a project called 'Oregon Health Priorities for the 1990s,' which involved nineteen community meetings (which were widely advertised with radio announcements, television advertisement, and direct mailings) across the state.[31] The set of criteria (for rationing health services) that was devised through this process of citizen interaction did not reflect an unquestionably fair distribution of health services, although it was consistent with trends that were emerging elsewhere which focus on preventive strategies.

The most important outcome of the community meetings organized by OHD was that a debate on social values and health care priorities was opened. 'Following the community meetings, in September 1988, 50 delegates (including 24 participants from the community meetings) met as a Citizen's Health Care Parliament.'[32] Delegates to the Citizen's Health Care Parliament tabled fifteen resolutions, the most important of which was that 'allocation of health resources should be based, in part, on a scale of public attitudes that quantifies the trade-off between length of life and quality of life. The full set of principles was then published and sent to all state legislators. Many of the principles established by the Health Care Parliament are now reflected in Oregon's Senate Bills 27 and 935.'[33] These examples of citizen initiative would guide the development and implementation of the Oregon Health Plan through several stages to its finalized form.

The first stage of the reform process involved ranking 1,600 condition–treatment pairs according to citizens' values (ascertained through a telephone survey) and technical criteria. The primary method used in the priority-setting exercise was cost–benefit analysis, which proved to be ineffective. This method of analysis led to a counterintuitive ordering of condition–treatment pairs. For example, crooked teeth received a higher ranking than early treatment for Hodgkin's disease, and dealing with thumbsucking ranked higher than hospitalization of a child for starvation.[34] Members of the commission, however, were not surprised, claiming that the first exercise was merely a test of the method. Cost-benefit analysis was quickly abandoned, as was the first list. Commission Chair Harvey Klevit said, 'I looked at the first two pages of that list and threw it in the trash can.'[35]

In the next attempt to rank order condition–treatment pairs, the commission relied more heavily on public values and clinical judgment. For example, Fox and Leichter explain:

> One widely debated issue ... was the relative priority assigned to various preventive medical and dental services. While some members of the commission ... felt that the high value assigned to preventive services by Oregonians in the community forums dictated that such services receive a high priority, some of the physician members were less convinced about the relative utility of, say, nutritional supplements and dental check-ups. In the end, however, the force of expressed community values prevailed, and preventive health services received a high priority on the list.[36]

The degree to which 'community values' ultimately prevailed remains, however, an open question. In 1992, President Bush's administration rejected Oregon's application for Medicaid waivers on the grounds that the process of community decision-making generated discriminatory results. Specifically, the administration was urged by the National Legal Center for the Medically Dependent and Disabled to reject the proposals because 'only some of the people surveyed were disabled [which meant that] the responses were likely to be prejudicial and reflect negative stereotypes about people with disabilities.'[37] Medicaid waivers were eventually granted by the Clinton administration, but only after clinical judgment had mitigated the effects of the community consultations.

System reform was not directly addressed during the Medicaid reform process (the private insurance, multi-payer system remains firmly in place). Nevertheless, institutional reforms were implemented, which might eventually lead, through incremental change, to a more equitable system. The engagement of citizens in the rationing exercise served to justify and legitimize the process, which was criticized for its lack of diversity, and its underrepresentation of low socioeconomic status groups. (As already noted, it was such participation that led, ultimately, to the rejection of Medicaid waivers by the Bush administration.) Those who attended the community meetings tended to be employed, educated, privately insured, middle-aged white women. According to Michael Brannigan: 'Over 69% of the participants were either health care or mental health workers; over 63% were women; an overwhelming number were insured (90.6%), and of these 4.4% were Medicaid recipients; 67% were college (university) graduates; 93% were white (the proportion of white adult Oregonians in the general population was 92%); and 34% had annual incomes of over US$50 000 (the average household income in the state was between US$24 000 and US$34 000).'[38]

By engaging the community in the Medicaid reform process in Oregon, legislators recognized that determining which services to fund and which citizens to include in the plan were value-laden decisions that should be made through a process of community-guided clinical judgment, rather than by technical experts, and in so doing were able to accord a significant degree of legitimacy to the rationing exercise. No other state has yet followed Oregon's lead in engaging citizens in a rationing experiment. There are, however, health decisions organizations in many states, as well as a national umbrella organization (American Health Decisions). Engaging citizens in decision-making is becoming part of the health policy landscape in North America.

The Politics of Participation

Having these North American experiences in mind, we may ask, What is it that the community governance structures will achieve? With yet another reorganization of health care governance structures in Nova Scotia, somewhat greater although limited success with the participatory exercise in Saskatchewan, and a community rationing exercise in Oregon that was marred by the discriminatory effects of citizen deliberation, there must be a strong political rationale for continuing to make community governance structures a priority on health care reform agendas. In some estimations, greater citizen inclusion in decision-making is 'a laudable goal in itself,' regardless of its institutional capabilities.[39] That community participation is inherently good is a claim that is, most likely, based on democratic appeal.

Democracy, Distribution, and Citizenship

One significant element of appeal for community governance structures is that, because they are included in decision-making processes concerning the redistribution of health care services, citizens can actively protect their perceived rights. The right to health care has been protected by the state in Canada for more than three decades, which means that citizens might have been well served, but not *empowered*, by such protection (i.e., their capacity for action has not increased). The possibilities for empowerment, in the context of current reform strategies, are questionable.

As explained, until very recently in Nova Scotia, the balance of power in the departmental structure was held by the non-designated organizations. Despite the reorganizational efforts of the Hamm government, amid the chaos of yet another restructuring effort, many elements of the system will remain constant. Physicians and institutions will continue to consume the vast proportion of resources, and coincident with that power, will direct future reform agendas. In addition, very little decision-making power will reside at the community level, which will undermine the effectiveness of community action directed at assessing needs and establishing community health plans.[40] Thus, citizens in Nova Scotia (as well as citizens in other provinces that have merely solicited citizen input) have been (and will continue to be) included in community decision-making processes but not empowered by them. Citizen input is not equivalent to citizen governance. It is the latter that has the potential to empower citizens by enabling them to actively protect their own rights and fulfil duties. Reform agendas for such initiatives in Saskatchewan, which have created citizen *governance* structures, are therefore more promising because that type of engagement promises to protect rights, aggregate interests, *and* empower citizens.

The question of whether community participation resulted in protection of rights and empowerment is somewhat less relevant in the Oregon case. In the United States, health care is not universally provided as a social right of citizenship. Community-based decision-making is not directed at protecting health care as a right, meaning health care is not a symbol of national identity *in addition to* being a set of important services. The degree to which citizens were empowered through the process in Oregon is, perhaps, a matter of perception. Citizens were invited to open political fora to share their opinions, ideas, and recommendations, which were tabled in reports that were frequently consulted by key decision-makers. Thus, while citizens formally played only an advisory role, their advice provided the foundation for the reformed system.

Lawrence Jacobs, Theodore Marmor, and Jonathan Oberlander, conclude that the most important function of democratic deliberation in the Oregon case was that of consensus-building.[41] Made possible by the state's participatory culture, the process

> offered reformers a political opportunity. Instead of experts designing OHP in a closed room, policy entrepreneurs chose a process that methodically sought out the attention of everyday Oregonians and sparked a very public debate across the state. Reformers solicited public participation as a part of a genuine effort to incorporate the public's 'substantive input on the relative importance of health care services.' But they also recognized the political benefits of public participation.[42]

Citizens in Oregon, through participating, came to understand the complexities of the process, and they could identify with the goals of reform. Surprisingly, the political justifications for, and developmental effects of, citizen deliberation might constitute the most important innovations and subsequent lessons of the Oregon rationing exercise, despite the attention attracted by 'the list.'[43] Community engagement as consensus-building was important because it provided a basis for political agreement among Democrats, Republicans, the Oregon Medical Association, and citizens' groups. Such broad agreement was instrumental in implementing the reforms and moving towards the goal of universal coverage (although the most important and ambitious step on the road to universality, the employer mandate, was repealed).[44]

How is this analysis relevant to Canadian experiences with community engagement in health care decision-making? How can Canadian health care reform efforts be evaluated within the well-developed debates[45] concerning deliberative democracy? As explained in Chapter 3, universally available health care services have become institutionalized as social rights of citizenship in Canada. This means that Canadians expect that the right to health care will be protected by the state. Canadians seem to be well beyond the need for deliberative processes aimed at securing universal entitlement. Those engaged in health care debate in Canada are arguing from tenuous universality, meaning that proposals for reform are considered (almost exclusively) within defences for maintaining the existing (universal) arrangements.

Canadians assume that justice requires an equal distribution of health resources in society; however, implicit rationing efforts in Canada threaten to undermine commitments to universality. Let us consider whether citizen participation can help reinforce these commitments that are purported to be essential not only for the health of the Canadian population, but for maintaining national identity.

Democratic Deliberation in Canada

Deliberative democracy for health care is aimed at protecting interests and developing consensus. In the Canadian context, the development of a certain civic-mindedness among the citizenry (translated as social rights identity, which indicates a sense of national pride and shared values) has already been achieved. Health care is Canada's most unifying national symbol. Canadians seem to agree that, as a matter of citizenship, each individual ought to be entitled to a comprehensive range of health services. Throughout the incremental process that resulted in the current health system, citizens came to consider universal health care to be a right. In Canada, social rights identity was developed during the creation and expansion of the health care system with strong political commitments. Hence, it seems counterintuitive to posit that the dismantling of hospital and medical insurance programs will further develop this type of civic-mindedness or consensus among Canadians.

Moreover, both the development and maintenance of social rights and participation in decision-making are directed at the goal of political equality. Health care in Canada is being transformed to embody competing theoretical justifications. On the one hand, health care in Canada is a social right, and as such, it seems to require nothing (other than proof of citizenship) from the claimant. On the other hand, Canadian provinces have created, or are in the process of creating, community governance structures in order to include citizens in decision-making concerning distributional equity. It will no longer be the case that Canadians are passively entitled to health services. Public health coverage will not become contingent on participation, but, as the structures develop, those who do participate will be responsible – morally, professionally, or both – for the impact of their decisions.

Social rights are a range of benefits to which each member of the political community is entitled as a matter of citizenship, are important not simply because governments ought to provide universal health care, subsidized education and housing, and the like, to mitigate the harsh effects of markets, but because the provision of these benefits enables citizens, regardless of social class, to fulfil certain duties as citizens. In Marshall's account, equality was defined passively: all citizens were equally entitled to receive benefits. Participation – which is also directed at the goal of political equality – clearly requires active citizenship. Thus, it seems that there are two competing theoretical justifications for equality in the Canadian health care system. Both should be thoroughly examined before reformers invest much more time, effort, and public resources into citizen-engagement exercises.

In spite of theoretical inconsistencies, however, it is possible that the competing theoretical justifications for equality are compatible, if not reinforcing. If the social rights thesis, as originally formulated, contains a reciprocal relationship between citizens and the state, a mutual exchange of entitlements and duties, then community-engagement exercises for health care might provide opportunities for citizens to fulfil their obligations of citizenship. The degree to which such participation could achieve substantive equality is open to debate.[46]

The Value of Participation

On the question of whether participation is inclusive or exclusive, there is no consensus. At first glance, it seems that participatory governance must be, by its very nature, more inclusive, empowering, and edifying than representative forms. This view, expounded by Jean-Jacques Rousseau, John Stuart Mill, and Carole Pateman, posits that by deliberating in their own affairs, citizens develop as human beings.

'The goal of politics is the transformation and education of the participants.'[47] Rousseau explains, in his treatise *The Social Contract*, that freedom in society is contingent on the participation of each individual in political, cultural, and economic affairs. Deliberation in the public sphere is necessary so that humans can cast off their chains and become citizens. In his *Letter to M. D'Alembert on the Theatre*, Rousseau explains that the theatre will lead to the degeneration of society in Geneva: 'It is there that they go to forget their friends, neighbors, and relations in order to concern themselves with fables, in order to cry for the misfortunes of the dead, or to laugh at the expense of the living.'[48] This removal of the individual from the immediate, collective concerns and duties of daily life is particularly troubling for Rousseau. He asks: 'What then does he go to see at the theatre? Precisely what he wants to find everywhere: lessons of virtue for the public, from which he excepts himself, and people sacrificing everything to their duty while nothing is exacted from him.'[49]

Full democratic citizenship consists of rights (namely, some secured freedom) and responsibilities or civic duties. In such an arrangement, participation in public affairs is essential. For Rousseau, citizens' participation in the community includes engagement in cultural as well as political activities. The theatre is threatening because it distracts people not only from matters of governance, and hence from gaining a civic education, but also from cultivating their own talents (playing music, telling stories).

Similarly, Pateman explains that democratic deliberation serves an important developmental or educative function: 'The major function of participation in the theory of participatory democracy is therefore an educative one, educative in the very widest sense, including both the psychological aspect and the gaining of practice in democratic skills and procedures.'[50] The indispensability of participation to a democracy affirms the alienability of human beings from their ideas and interests. Recreating discursive fora in advanced democracies is particularly important, given the unparalleled distractions and alienating effects of the technological age.

Notwithstanding the practical difficulties in encouraging and supporting participation, even in the widest sense, it is not a foregone conclusion that participatory or 'active' citizenship translates into positive political inclusion. Jane Mansbridge explains that by insisting on equality in participatory fora, diversity is not adequately respected and the creative process is impoverished:

Beyond a certain point in any process, attempts to ensure absolutely equal power in every decision will reduce output. The higher the value one puts on the benefits of equal respect, political education and equal protection, the higher the price one will be willing to pay in output. Many participatory democrats are willing to reduce the quantity and perhaps also the quality of production quite dramatically in order to increase equality. Responding to Isaiah Berlin's example of a symphony, some participatory democrats would certainly argue that if the roles of conductor and players could not be rotated or the prestige of the jobs made more equal, the musicians should consider playing music that does not require a conductor, such as chamber music or some forms of jazz.[52]

Thus, inclusive decision-making exercises threaten to level-down the quality of diverse experiences and skills that each participant brings to the deliberative forum.

Lynn Sanders goes on to argue 'against deliberation' for similar reasons.[52] Taking aim at advocates of deliberation,[53] Sanders argues that the internal dynamics of mutual respect and equality, which are necessary preconditions for legitimate deliberation, cannot be achieved. Yet Sanders seems to gloss over the most obvious problem with deliberative fora, namely, that not all citizens will choose to, or be able to, participate.

This most obvious problem, recognized by Joshua Cohen and Joel Rogers, suggests that mere possibilities for participation are not sufficient.[54] However, the argument might be made that opportunities for participation are akin to voting: not everyone votes, although every eligible citizen has the right to do so (therefore 'the vote' itself is positive and empowering, regardless of who actually votes). Similarly, opportunities for participation would change the nature of politics, afford greater possibilities for inclusion or diversity, regardless of who actually participates in meetings.

Far fewer people will participate in community governance structures than will vote. Moreover, the current constitution and rationale for structures do not foster proper dynamics for inclusion. In sum, until further consideration is given to the competing justifications (which is beyond the scope of this project), it will be theoretically and practically difficult to square social rights (passive) with participatory (active) citizenship. More will be said about this problem and what might be done to remedy it in a subsequent section.

Parliamentary Governance and Democracy

Another factor contributes to stasis. Executive domination of policy processes in a parliamentary system of government results in a relatively small public sphere. Because governmental authority is concentrated in a single decision-making body (cabinet), possibilities are diminished for competing domains of popular authority. In contradistinction, the congressional system of government allows for, and perhaps necessitates, a considerable degree of citizen involvement in political decision-making, which greatly increases the size of the public sphere.

The incongruence of an open deliberative forum (many voices) and a parliamentary system of government (two voices: government and opposition) indicates the theoretical difficulty of the former in the context of the latter. However, the limitations of the executive system make participation all the more important.

As the primary cause of death changed from communicable to non-communicable disease, the responsibility of each individual for his or her own health grew (this was explained in some detail in Chapter 6). It is no longer the case that state action in health care (exclusively) can significantly contribute to better overall health indicators. Responsibility-taking is not merely a right-wing strategy for cost containment, but a matter of practical importance, and consonant with Marshall's citizenship equation (rights + duties = citizenship).

Evaluation

If debate is necessary as part of a plan to move beyond stasis, is purposeful debate in community governance structures for health care possible? The lesson to be taken from the Oregon experience is that citizen participation does shape public policy and that such participation can be both empowering and discriminatory. On the one hand, citizen engagement (either as input or governance) may be important in the Canadian case to build consensus (as in Oregon), at least in recognition of problems. The degree to which viable solutions can be drafted, on the other hand, is much more doubtful. As in the Oregon case, members of community governance structures in Canadian provinces are 'largely middle-aged, well educated and well off.'[55] The potential for such an unrepresentative group to make unrepresentative (if not discriminatory) decisions, is great.

Let us also revisit the question that was set in Chapter 2: Is this what Marshall had in mind? Is it consistent with Marshall's vision of citizenship? To the former question, the answer is likely negative. Marshall did not envision that citizens would help to determine their own social rights. This was the responsibility of the state. The answer to the latter question, however, is affirmative. Participation is consistent with Marshall's conception of citizenship as a reciprocal arrangement between citizens and the state. Perhaps participation could best be employed to build consensus regarding problems and limitations, rather than to set priorities for health care reform.

A Solution? Citizenship, Entitlement, and Differentiation

The promise of community governance structures is that communities will be able, through the processes of deliberation and decision-making, to build up their own identities and have these identities reflected in patterns of entitlement and service delivery. If the community health board in north Halifax, for example, is representative of a large proportion of people of colour, or elderly persons suffering with respiratory disorders, then suggestions can be made so that policy is responsive to those communities.

The problem, however, is finding ways to have the community health board reflect the community it represents. As the Oregon experience shows, and is revealed by the information gathered by Jonathan Lomas, Gerry Veenstra, and John Woods on regional governance structures in Canada, not all segments of a community are represented, and those who do participate tend to be from particular cohorts.[56] Even if communities were fully representative, they are geographically determined, and they do not necessarily reflect the communities of people that a differentiated approach ought to address. Simon Watney, building on Ralf Dahrendorf's ideas, explains that in the British context, it needs to be recognized that

> entitlements must be sufficiently flexible to be able to respond to the emergence of *new* social identities and constituencies. Citizenship thus stands to unite the overlapping interests of individuals and groups whose self-conscious identities are specific to the postwar period, whether in relation to race, gender, sexuality, disability, or whatever. The concept of citizenship is sensitive to the fact that our identities are multiple and

mobile, that we all increasingly identify ourselves with aspects of race, class, sexuality and so on, in ways that are idiosyncratic and subject to frequent change over time.[57]

The argued inability of the party system in Great Britain to recognize these multiple identities presents a serious obstacle to reform, and an affront to citizenship. This critique also applies to Canada. Marshall's caveat that citizenship is an evolving concept, would support this movement towards reconceptualizing citizenship.

Thus, community governance structures, as currently constituted, are problematic in that they are likely to reproduce discriminatory effects, as happened in Oregon. Stigmatized groups, such as HIV/AIDS patients, might be worse off with community governance structures. Yet, community governance structures are an important compo nent of provincial reform agendas, and they have great potential for addressing the gaps in electoral and party politics – rather than replicating them.

What, then, are the options? There are two changes that might be made to harness the positive potential of community governance structures. First, community meetings could be organized to address narrow and well-defined issues. For example, one open public meeting might address HIV/AIDS issues, another might address seniors and pharmaceuticals, or home care options. This would bring interested and affected parties to the meetings, who might not attend general community meetings. Here the problem, again, as evidenced in Oregon with Medicaid reform, is that people do not always choose to become involved in community decision-making exercises, even when the issues clearly affect them.

Second, ad hoc representative boards should be established. Some balance has been achieved in most provinces with provincial appointments to regional health boards. However, the diversity that can be reflected in these permanent boards remains limited. Thus, regional and community health boards might have their mandates changed and clarified so that they function as advisory boards whose primary duty is to assemble ad hoc representative groups from the community to attend issue-oriented meetings. This second option would actually blend both suggestions, remedy the existing problems of improper representation of 'communities,' and eliminate the current practice of regional and community health boards producing unfocused 'wish lists' for reform.[58]

Conclusion

The rhetoric of grassroots initiatives, citizen inclusion, and community participation, in addition to the actual changes heralded by community-engagement exercises, have begun to adjust citizens' expectations about the role of the state. This allows governments in Canada to indirectly address issues of distributional equity at the same time that they dodge politically charged issues. Such developments are problematic. They demonstrate a glaring disregard for the theoretical and practical difficulties that result from competing justifications concerning equality (social rights versus participation) and from introducing fora for the exercise of popular authority in an executive-driven system.

To dismiss community-engagement exercises entirely, however, is to misconstrue the full intention of the social rights thesis and the unique opportunities that community governance structures potentially afford. Duties are not just the preserve of new right theorizing.[59] As explained in the preceding chapters, Canada is entering a fourth stage of social citizenship development that requires a new blend of individual responsibility-taking and collective entitlement. The social rights thesis asserts the latter, while some aspects of provincial reform agendas, notably community governance structures, have the potential to institutionalize the former. Unfortunately, it seems that the social rights thesis, at the same time that it protects collective entitlement, precludes important political initiatives aimed at individual responsibility-taking. The question remains, How can the right to health care be protected at the same time that stasis is attenuated?

8

Conclusion: Health Care and Universality – Looking Ahead

To the question of how to attenuate stasis while protecting entitlement, there is no definitive answer. Nevertheless, the analysis presented in this book is intended to provide some foundational support for understanding the right to health care and the need for moving beyond the social rights stage of policy and citizenship development. The evolution of rights discourse over the post–Second World War decades, as it applies to health care in Canada, reveals both individual and collective elements of entitlement. The enduring collective element is distinctly premodern, within the normative realm of discourse. The individualistic trend can be attributed to several forces pulling in the same direction: the Canadian Charter of Rights and Freedoms, the New Public Management, the Canada Health Act, the transition in the epidemiological contours of disease, and, as always, the influence of U.S. culture on Canadian political, economic, and social life.

The result, the beginning of a new blend of individual responsibility-taking and collective entitlement, may indicate that Canada is entering a fourth stage of citizenship development. The period of social rights development, of particular importance in the Canadian context, enabled the institutionalization of relatively generous patterns of entitlement to public health care. The practical benefits and symbolic value of such entitlement have resulted in the popular assertion that health care is a right of citizenship, and, as such, ought not to be significantly altered by governments trying to manage health care costs or reform health care systems. However, as demonstrated throughout this work, such defences of the right to health care have led to untenable positions and static conditions, and these continue to present serious problems.

The problems particular to Canadian health care are endemic to social rights theorizing generally. In Chapters 2 and 3 it was argued that the social rights thesis is outdated. The changing nature of social rights, in accordance with T.H. Marshall's claim that citizenship is an evolving concept, requires vigilant reconsideration and revision. Health care, Canada's most revered social entitlement program, was certainly one of Marshall's intended components of full social citizenship. However, Marshall's analysis pertained directly to issues of education and poverty in Great Britain. Modifications and specifications needed to be made to import Marshall's social rights analysis into the specific case of health care in Canada. Furthermore, Marshall's analysis was intended to address a specific period in time, and, necessarily, a certain set of circumstances that were characteristic of that period.

In Chapter 6 I explored the connections between socioeconomic status and health. The epidemiological transition reveals that income disparity in a society has a direct impact on the health of that society and that health ought to be a priority not just of individuals, but of their societies. The shift in the main causes of death, from communicable to non-communicable diseases, implicates social factors. This means that in contrast to the public health measures that were necessary to stem the epidemics of the nineteenth and early twentieth centuries, a new type of collective concern for health is needed to address diseases linked to the distribution of income and status within societies.

The right to health care in the 1940s translated as the expectation that communicable diseases would be brought under control and that a range of advanced medical services would be available for private consumption. In the 1950s and 1960s the right to health care began to indicate an expectation that health services would be distributed as public goods. By the end of the 1970s, health care had become part of Canada's collective conscience – and protecting the right against retrenchment was a matter of practical concern, as well as national identity.

Social class is still a primary source of inequality. However, it is important to recognize that inequality is not one-dimensional: social class intersects with ascriptive and acquired characteristics to produce disparate levels of health status and access to health care services. Thus, citizenship in Canada requires respect for multiple sources of inequality, as they intersect with socioeconomic status. Differences based on language, gender, sexual orientation, ability, and race make necessary increasingly flexible policy responses. Universal health care coverage aims to ensure that poor people have access to medical services. In addition, health insurance should address other, perhaps even more complex communities.

Defences of the right to health care invariably address Canadian values. How Canadians consent to provide health care services to one another is indicative of how they believe they ought to treat one another concerning different social, political, and even constitutional matters, and in other parts of the globe. In other areas of Canadian social policy, this spirit of generosity is replaced with a chary disposition. Thus, health care policy in Canada demands scholarly attention because of the puzzle that it presents: the right to health care in Canada is paradigmatic of Canadian culture, but is also an enigmatic social democratic covenant. Universal health care seems to be definitive of Canadian identity, while at the same time it is a special case.

Beyond Stasis: Identity Rights as Citizenship Development

The foregoing analysis suggests that Canada has entered a fourth stage of citizenship development. This assertion has clear links to, and implications for, legal rights claiming. The Charter's commitments to 'categorical equity' have been able to protect, if not assert, differences based on gender, sexuality, language, and ability. Such commitments provide evidence for a more active and inclusive era of citizenship.

This new era of identity rights and differentiated citizenship has implications for health care. As demonstrated in Chapters 3 and 4, health care is increasingly defended in the language of rights. The right to health care, as an essential component of Canadian citizenship, has come to embody a new blend of individual responsibility-taking and collective entitlement that might be relevant to other areas of concern, even if the dynamics of health policy (and the apparent generosity that they engender) are not representative of other Canadian policy fields.

Movement beyond stasis and towards more active and inclusive models of Canadian citizenship can be discerned in provincial health care reform agendas. As argued in Chapter 7, community governance fora give structure to a reciprocal arrangement between citizens and the state. As the state continues to deal with, and fund accordingly, new patterns of disease, care, and entitlement, citizens can fulfil their duties by engaging in decision-making processes. The flexibility that is potentially afforded by these models is enormous. The possibility that these models will become institutionalized or effective is, at best, indistinct.

Effective approaches to dealing with general issues of health care and entitlement must be found, so that prospects for dealing with the more acute dynamics of inequality, epidemiology, and citizenship might be improved. In particular, it is important to understand the meaning of the right to health care and the direction of citizenship development as it pertains to health care, in order to deal with those citizens who are members of groups that have much different experiences with access to medically necessary services (stigmatized populations, including AIDS patients and the mentally ill), that is, groups that are differentially entitled and particularly dependent on services that fall outside the parameters of the general public plan.

Such an approach should include a commitment to what the World Health Organization calls 'new universalism.' Contemporary WHO values 'lead away from a form of universalism that has governments attempting to provide and finance everything for everybody. This "classical" universalism, although seldom advanced in extreme form, shaped the formation of many European health systems. It achieved important successes. But classical universalism fails to recognize both resource limits and the limits of government.'[1] In its place the WHO advocates a '"new universalism," that recognizes governments' limits but retains government responsibility for the leadership and finance of health systems.'[2] Under this rubric it might be possible to develop ancillary programs like pharmacare and home care, although, as explained in Chapter 5, the mercurial dynamics of federal–provincial relations will ultimately determine the feasibility of any new programs.

It is also imperative that such an approach addresses citizen engagement. The decline of the welfare state and the unreliability of the social rights thesis make necessary the consideration of the inclusion of citizens in decision-making processes, even if prospects in some if not all Canadian contexts are less than ideal. However, clarifications will have to be made regarding the goals of participatory exercises. Will citizens be making decisions or merely advising? Are the issues to be negotiated discrete and well defined, or will participants be contemplating the broadest issues at hand? Can social rights be protected at the same time that diversity is accommodated and decision-making is made more inclusive?

The right to health care has been for Canada a source of both pride and stasis. Health care is a vital social program, but, despite its popularity as a symbol of Canada's social superiority to the United States, it is not beyond reproach. As citizenship develops beyond the social rights stage, there is increasing dissonance in rights claiming for health care, the nature of entitlement, and the provision of services. The complexity of the burgeoning range of pressures for change makes solutions to 'crises' of funding and entitlement both pressing and elusive. Defending the right to health care against all encroachments does not seem to be an appropriate or sophisticated response to complex problems.

As progress is made towards the goal of universality in the United States, the challenge of difference will facilitate the movement towards health care coverage for the entire population (although this is likely to be done in a very piecemeal way), rather than stymie it (as was the case in the 1960s; the tumultuous civil rights era effectively pre-empted the development of social rights). In Canada, the challenge of difference offers a way out of social rights stasis at the same time that it offers to revise and secure universality.

The Canadian universal health care system, the perennial model for North American health care reform, has become the target of much criticism at the same time that it remains beyond reproach. Continued defences of the right to health care cannot by themselves secure access and entitlement for all Canadians. What is needed, instead, is an evaluation of how vulnerable groups fare in the current health care system,[3] recognition of the multiplicity of differentiated citizenship claims across the country, an understanding of how these claims can be expressed and accommodated in public policy, and a strategy for identity-based communities informing and interacting with geographically based entities.

Notes

1 Introduction

1 Will Kymlicka and Wayne Norman, 'Return of the Citizen: A Survey of Recent Work on Citizenship Theory,' in Ronald Beiner, ed., *Theorizing Citizenship* (Albany: State University of New York Press, 1995).

2 Iris Marion Young, *Justice and the Politics of Difference* (Princeton: Princeton University Press, 1990). Will Kymlicka, *Multicultural Citizenship: A Liberal Theory of Minority Rights* (Oxford: Oxford University Press, 1996). Will Kymlicka and Wayne Norman, eds., *Citizenship in Diverse Societies* (Oxford: Oxford University Press, 2000). Charles Taylor, 'Multiculturalism and "the Politics of Recognition,"' in Amy Gutmann, ed., *Multiculturalism: Examining the Politics of Recognition* (Princeton: Princeton University Press, 1994). Michael Sandel, *Democracy's Discontent: America in Search of a Public Philosophy* (Cambridge, Mass.: Harvard University Press, 1996). James Tully, *Strange Multiplicity: Constitutionalism in an Age of Diversity* (Cambridge: Cambridge University Press, 1995).

3 Kymlicka and Norman, 'Return of the Citizen,' 302, 306.

4 Richard Wilkinson, 'The Epidemiological Transition: From Material Scarcity to Social Disadvantage,' *Daedalus*, Fall 1994, 61–78. Paul Farmer, *Infections and Inequalities: The Modern Plagues* (Berkeley: University of California Press, 1999). Robert G. Evans, Morris Barer, and Theodore Marmor, eds., *Why Are Some People Healthy and Others Not? Determinants of Health of Populations* (New York: De Gruyter, 1994).

5 Evans, Barer, Marmor, *Why Are Some People Healthy?*

6 Quoted in ibid., 3.

7 Quoted in Farmer, *Infections and Inequalities*, 15.

8 Ibid.

9 Young, *Justice and the Politics of Difference*.
10 Kymlicka and Norman, 'Return of the Citizen.'
11 Ibid.
12 T.H. Marshall, *Class, Citizenship and Social Development* (New York: Double-day, 1964).
13 Allen Schick, 'Budgetary Adaptations to Resource Scarcity,' in Charles Levine and Irene Rubin, eds., *Fiscal Stress and Public Policy* (London: Sage, 1980).

2 Health Care Entitlement and Citizenship Development

1 Canadian Federation of Agriculture quoted in Malcolm Taylor, *Health Insurance and Canadian Public Policy: The Seven Decisions That Created the Canadian Health Insurance System* (Montreal: McGill-Queen's University Press, 1987), 33.
2 Ibid., 80.
3 Canada, Health Canada, Speaking notes for the Hon. Alan Rock, Minister of Health at the 130th Annual Meeting of the Canadian Medical Association, Victoria, BC, 20 August, 1997.
4 For defences of the social rights thesis, see Desmond King and Jeremy Waldron, 'Citizenship, Social Citizenship and the Defence of Welfare Provision,' *British Journal of Political Science* 18 (1988), 415–43. Gosta Esping-Andersen, 'Power and Distributional Regimes,' *Politics and Society* 14 (1985), 223–56. Kathi Friedman, *Legitimation of Social Rights and the Western Welfare State* (Chapel Hill: University of North Carolina Press, 1981). Julie Parker, *Social Policy and Citizenship* (London: Macmillan, 1975). Ralf Dahrendorf, *The Modern Social Conflict: An Essay on the Politics of Liberty* (New York: Weidenfeld and Nicolson, 1988), chapters 7 and 8. Dahrendorf, 'The Changing Quality of Citizenship,' in Bart van Steenbergen, ed., *The Condition of Citizenship* (London: Sage, 1994).
5 Alan Maslove, 'Time to Fold or Up the Ante: The Federal Role in Health Care,' John F. Graham Memorial Lecture, Dalhousie University, 9 March 1995; Thomas Courchene, *ACCESS: A Convention on the Canadian Economic and Social Systems*. Working Paper prepared for the Ministry of Intergovernmental Affairs, Government of Ontario. Reprinted in *Assessing Access: Towards a New Social Union, Proceedings on the Symposium on the Courchene Proposal*. Institute of Intergovernmental Relations (Kingston: Queen's University, 1996).
6 Canada, Health Canada, *National Health Expenditures in Canada 1975–1996*, Policy and Consultation Branch, June 1997, 2. See also Canadian Institute for Health Information (CIHI) and Statistics Canada, *Health Care in Canada:*

A First Annual Report (2000), 17. The Canadian Institutes for Health Information (CIHI) and Statistics Canada report that the public share of total health expenditures is expected to rise slightly in 1999 and 2000. See CIHI and Statistics Canada, *Health Care in Canada 2001*, 72, www.cihi.ca.

7   U.S. Department of Health and Human Services, Health Care Financing Administration, *Health Care Financing Review* 17 (Spring) (1996), 229. Public expenditures for health care represent approximately 6.6 per cent and 6.8 per cent GDP for the United States and Canada, respectively. World Bank, *World Development Report: Knowledge for Development 1998/99* (1999), table 7, 202–3.

8   Richard Kronick and Todd Gilmer, 'Explaining the Decline in Health Insurance Coverage, 1979–1995,' *Health Affairs* 18/2 (1999), 43.

9   Miriam Smith, 'Retrenching the Sacred Trust: Medicare and Canadian Federalism,' in François Rocher and Miriam Smith, eds., *New Trends in Canadian Federalism* (Peterborough: Broadview Press, 1995).

10 Lawrence Mead, 'Citizenship and Social Policy: T.H. Marshall and Poverty,' *Social Philosophy and Policy* 14/2 (1997), 197–230.

11 Mead, 'Citizenship and Social Policy,' 203.

12 Ibid.

13 Ibid.

14 T.H. Marshall, *Class, Citizenship and Social Development* (New York: Doubleday, 1964), 78.

15 Ibid.

16 Allen Schick, 'Budgetary Adaptations to Resource Scarcity,' in Charles Levine and Irene Rubin, eds., *Fiscal Stress and Public Policy* (London: Sage, 1980).

17 Arthur Dyck, *Rethinking Rights and Responsibilities: The Moral Bonds of Community* (Cleveland: Pilgrim Press, 1994), 308.

18 See, e.g., Iris Marion Young, 'Polity and Group Difference: A Critique of the Ideal of Universal Citizenship,' *Ethics* 99 (1989), 250–74.

19 The essay and reprinted as chapter 4 in Marshall, *Class, Citizenship and Social Development*; the quotation is found on p. 76.

20 Ibid., 78.

21 Ibid.

22 Ibid., 103.

23 Jytte Klausen, 'Social Rights Advocacy and State Building: T.H. Marshall in the Hands of Social Reformers,' *World Politics* 47/2 (January 1995), 245.

24 Carolyn Hughes Tuohy, *Accidental Logics: The Dynamics of Change in the Health Care Arena in the United States, Britain and Canada* (New York: Oxford University Press, 1999), chapter 1.

25 J.M. Barbalet, *Citizenship: Rights, Struggle and Class Inequality* (Minneapolis: University of Minnesota Press, 1988).

26 Bryan Turner, ed., *Citizenship and Social Theory* (London: Sage, 1993). Barry Hindness, 'Citizenship and the Modern West,' in Bryan Turner, ed., *Citizenship and Social Theory* (London: Sage, 1993).
27 King and Waldron, 'Citizenship, Social Citizenship and the Defence of Welfare Provision.'
28 Marshall, *Class, Citizenship and Social Development*, 82.
29 Young, *'Polity and Group Difference.'*
30 Young's position as explained by Kymlicka and Norman, 'Return of the Citizen,' 303.

3 The Evolution of Social Rights in Canada

1 Katherine Graham and Susan Phillips, 'Citizen Engagement: Beyond the Customer Revolution,' *Canadian Public Administration* 40/2 (Summer 1990), 257.
2 Ibid.
3 Ibid.
4 Ibid.
5 Allen Schick, 'Budgetary Adaptations to Resource Scarcity,' in Charles Levine and Irene Rubin, eds., *Fiscal Stress and Public Policy* (London: Sage, 1980).
6 Malcolm Taylor, *Health Insurance and Canadian Public Policy: The Seven Decisions That Created the Canadian Health Insurance System* (Montreal and Kingston: McGill-Queen's University Press, 1987), 33.
7 This point is debatable. Public health insurance was considered initially at the federal level by Mackenzie King in 1919. It is with the Report of the Rowell-Sirois Commission that momentum towards publicly insured hospital and medical insurance began to build.
8 Donald Smiley, ed., *The Rowell-Sirois Report Abridged* (Toronto: McClelland and Stewart, 1964), 5.
9 Harley Dickinson, 'The Struggle for State Health Insurance: Reconsidering the Role of Saskatchewan Farmers,' *Studies in Political Economy* 41 (Summer 1993), 137–8.
10 Paul Barker, 'The Development of Major Shared-Cost Programs in Canada,' in R.D. Olling and M.W. Westmacott, eds., *Perspectives on Canadian Federalism* (Scarborough, Ont.: Prentice-Hall, 1988), 201.
11 Following the Second World War, the federal government made several proposals for public health insurance (Green Book Proposals, 1945). However, at this time the federal government was in a very strong position vis-à-vis the provinces, and was not compelled to act on the proposals. By 1957

the balance of power shifted and the federal government recognized its role in hospital insurance. Taylor, *Health Insurance and Canadian Public Policy* 78.

12 Malcolm Taylor, Michael Stevenson, and Paul Williams, *Medical Perspectives on Canadian Medicare: Attitudes of Canadian Physicians to Policies and Problems of the Medical Care Insurance Program* (Toronto: Institute for Behavioural Research, 1984), 3.

13 Ibid.

14 Ibid., 4.

15 Ibid., 5.

16 Ibid.

17 Ibid., 6.

18 Emmett Hall, *The Royal Commission on Health Services*, Report of the Hall Commission (Ottawa: R. Duhamel, Queen's Printer, 1964).

19 Ibid., 1, 28.

20 Ibid., 10.

21 Ibid., 4.

22 C.E.S. Franks, *The Parliament of Canada* (Toronto: University of Toronto Press, 1987), 7.

23 Health Charter for Canadians in *Hall Commission* vol. 1, 11–12. Emmett Hall, *The Royal Commission on Health Services* (Report) (Ottawa: R. Duhamel, Queen's Printer, 1964).

24 Paul Barker, 'The Development of Major Shared-Cost Programs in Canada,' in R.D. Olling and M.W. Westmacott, eds., *Perspectives on Canadian Federalism* (Scarborough: Prentice-Hall, 1988), 205.

25 Ibid., 207.

26 See Marion G. Wrobel, *The Federal Deficit and Universality of Social Programs* (Ottawa: Library of Parliament, Economics Division, 1989).

27 See Canada, Department of Finance, Budget 1999, *Building Today for a Better Tomorrow: Federal Financial Support for the Provinces and Territories*, 15 February, chart 3.

28 Jon Pierre, 'The Marketization of the State: Citizens, Consumers and the Emergence of the Public Market,' in B. Guy Peters and Donald Savoie, eds., *Governance in a Changing Environment* (Montreal and Kingston: McGill-Queen's University Press, 1995).

29 Ibid., 60.

30 Patricia O'Reilly, *Health Care Practitioners* (Toronto: University of Toronto Press, 2000), 57.

31 Pierre, 'The Marketization of the State,' 60.

32 Ibid.

33 Raymond Bazowski, 'Canadian Political Thought,' in James Bickerton and Alain Gagnon, eds., *Canadian Politics* (Peterborough: Broadview, 1995), 103.
34 Charles Taylor cited in ibid., 105.
35 Reg Whitaker, 'Rights in a Free and Democratic Society: Abortion,' in David Shugarman and Reg Whitaker, eds., *Federalism and Political Community* (Peterborough: Broadview, 1989), 327.
36 *Eldridge* v. *British Columbia (Attorney General)*, [1997] 3 S.C.R. 624.
37 See Colleen Flood, 'The Structure and Dynamics of Canada's Health Care System,' in J. Downie and T. Caulfield, eds., *Canadian Health Law and Policy* (Toronto: Butterworth, 1999), 5–50. *Cameron* v *Nova Scotia (A.G.)* (1997), 163 N.S.R. (2d) 391, 487 A.P.R. 391 (S.C.). See also *Waldman* v *Medical Services Commission of British Columbia*, 30 July 1997, Supreme Court of British Columbia, Docket numbers A952722, A961607. In this case, medical doctors in British Columbia challenged the constitutional validity of government limitations placed on their freedom to practise in 'overserviced' urban locations.
38 Marcia Rioux, 'Appropriate Uses of Law in Health Policy: Three Views, in Margaret A. Somerville, ed., *Do We Care? Renewing Canada's Commitment to Health* (Montreal: McGill-Queen's University Press, 1999), 147.
39 Ibid.
40 Ibid.
41 Will Kymlicka and Wayne Norman, 'Return of the Citizen: A Survey of Recent Work on Citizenship Theory,' in Ronald Beiner, ed., *Theorizing Citizenship* (Albany: SUNY Press, 1995), 301–2.
42 See Carolyn Tuohy, 'Medicine and the State in Canada: The Extra-Billing Issue in Perspective,' *Canadian Journal of Political Science* 21 (1988).
43 Raisa Deber, 'The Use and Misuse of Economics,' in Margaret A. Somerville, ed., *Do We Care? Renewing Canada's Commitment to Health* (Montreal: McGill-Queen's University Press, 1999).
44 Ibid., 63.

4 The Right to Health Care

1 Pat and Hugh Armstrong offer an excellent treatment of the 'crisis' of Canadian health care from a political economy perspective in *Wasting Away: The Undermining of Canadian Health Care* (Toronto: Oxford University Press, 1996). The Armstrongs' argument is based on several assumptions derived from the social rights thesis, but does not systematically challenge them.
2 T.H. Marshall, *Class, Citizenship and Social Development* (New York: Doubleday, 1964).

3 See Will Kymlicka, *Multicultural Citizenship: A Liberal Theory of Minority Rights* (Oxford: Oxford University Press, 1996). James Tully, *Strange Multiplicity: Constitutionalism in an Age of Diversity* (Cambridge: Cambridge University Press, 1995). Charles Taylor, 'Multiculturalism and the "Politics of Recognition,"' in Amy Gutmann, ed., *Multiculturalism: Examining the Politics of Recognition* (Princeton: Princeton University Press, 1994).

4 See, e.g., the Canadian Federation of Agriculture statement of 1942 quoted in Malcolm Taylor, *Health Insurance and Canadian Public Policy: The Seven Decisions That Created the Canadian Health Insurance System* (Montreal: McGill-Queen's University Press, 1987), 33: 'the people are thinking of health as a right of citizenship, of even greater importance than education or police protection, which are taken for granted.'

5 See Desmond King and Jeremy Waldron, 'Citizenship, Social Citizenship and the Defence of Welfare Provision,' *British Journal of Political Science* 18 (1988), 415–43. Gosta Esping-Andersen, 'Power and Distributional Regimes, *Politics and Society* 14 (1985), 223–56. Kathi Friedman, *Legitimation of Social Rights and the Western Welfare State* (Chapel Hill: UNC Press, 1981). Julie Parker, *Social Policy and Citizenship* (London: Macmillan, 1975). Ralf Dahrendorf, *The Modern Social Conflict: An Essay on the Politics of Liberty* (New York: Weidenfeld and Nicolson, 1988), chapters 7 and 8. Lawrence Mead, 'Citizenship and Social Policy: T.H. Marshall and Poverty,' *Journal of Social Philosophy and Policy* 14 (1997). Joe Soss, 'Welfare Provision, Civil Society, and Democracy in the United States,' paper prepared for The World Project on Civil Society Author's Conference, Center for the Study of Voluntary Organizations and Service, Washington, DC, 3–4 June 1999.

6 Carolyn Tuohy, 'Social Policy: Two Worlds,' in Michael Atkinson, ed., *Governing Canada: Institutions and Public Policy* (Toronto: Harcourt Brace Jovanovich, 1993).

7 H.L.A. Hart, 'Are There Any Natural Rights?' in David Lyons, ed., *Rights* (Belmont: Wadsworth, 1979), 14.

8 Ibid., 19.

9 Ibid., 15.

10 It is possible that the use of general taxation revenues to fund universally distributed social goods is 'coercive.' This is an important argument, yet well beyond the scope of this chapter. See Robert Nozick, *Anarchy, State, and Utopia* (Oxford: Basil Blackwell, 1974).

11 Hart, 'Are There Any Natural Rights?' 15.

12 Joel Feinberg, 'The Nature and Value of Rights,' in David Lyons, ed., *Rights* (Belmont: Wadsworth, 1979), 78.

13 Hart, 'Are There Any Natural Rights?' 14.

14 Feinberg, 'The Nature and Value of Rights,' 80.
15 Robert Young, 'Dispensing With Moral Rights,' *Political Theory* 6 (1978), 63. See also Ronald Beiner, *What's the Matter with Liberalism?* (Berkeley and Los Angeles: University of California Press, 1992), chapter 4.
16 Feinberg, *'The Nature and Value of Rights,'* 87.
17 See Ronald Dworkin, *Foundations of Liberal Equality,* Tanner Lectures on Human Values XI (Salt Lake City: University of Utah Press, 1990).
18 Ronald Dworkin, *Taking Rights Seriously* (London: Duckworth, 1978).
19 Richard Tuck, *Natural Rights Theories: Their Origin and Development* (Cambridge: Cambridge University Press, 1979), 1.
20 Ibid., 8.
21 Arthur Dyck, *Rethinking Rights and Responsibilities: The Moral Bonds of Community* (Cleveland: Pilgrim Press, 1994), 311.
22 Richard G. Wilkinson explains that cancer, stroke, and heart disease are social diseases, linked, among other environmental factors, to social disparities within populations. The 'transition from the primacy of material constraints to social constraints as the limiting condition on the quality of human life,' generalizes current epidemiological patterns. In other words, health is a factor of relative inequality within a society, rather than relative inequality among societies. Richard G. Wilkinson, 'The Epidemiological Transition: From Material Scarcity to Social Disadvantage,' *Daedalus*, Fall 1994, 65.
23 Thomas Paine, 'Agrarian Justice,' in Philip S. Foner, ed., *The Complete Writings of Thomas Paine* (New York: The Citadel Press, 1945), 610. Originally published in 1796.
24 Ibid., 612–13.
25 Ibid., 620.
26 C.B. Macpherson, *The Political Theory of Possessive Individualism* (Oxford: Clarendon Press, 1962).
27 Michael Hayes and Sholom Glouberman, 'Population Health, Sustainable Development and Policy Future,' Canadian Policy Research Networks Discussion Paper, H/01, September 1999, 9.
28 See Emmett Hall, *The Royal Commission on Health Services* (Report) (Ottawa: R. Duhamel, Queen's Printer, 1964), 1, 28.

5 Sources of Stasis: Budgeting, Perceptions of Privatization, and the Politics of Federalism

 1 World Health Organization, *The World Health Report: Making a Difference* (Geneva: WHO 1999), 37.

2 See David Naylor, 'Evidence-Based Health Care: A Reality Check,' Amyot Lecture delivered at Health Canada, Tunney's Pasture, Ottawa, Ontario, 18 October 2000 (www.hc-sc.gc.ca/english/amyot2000_5.htm).

3 Kaiser Family Foundation, *Medicaid and the Uninsured*, May 2000, www.kff.org/content/2000/1420 (site visited on 3 June, 2001).

4 See James Morone, *The Democratic Wish: Popular Participation and the Limits of American Government* (New Haven: Yale University Press, 1990), 285.

5 See Abraham Verghese, *My Own Country: A Doctor's Story* (New York: Vintage Books, 1995).

6 Marginal entitlement zones refer to ambiguities in patterns of entitlement to health services for segments of the population.

7 See Simon Watney, 'Practices of Freedom: "Citizenship" and the Politics of Identity in the Age of AIDS,' in John Rutherford, ed., *Identity: Community, Culture and Difference* (New York: New York University Press, 1990).

8 See Carolyn Hughes Tuohy, *Accidental Logics: The Dynamics of Change in the Health Care Arena in the United States, Britain and Canada* (New York: Oxford University Press, 1999). Tuohy, 'Conflict and Accommodation in the Canadian Health Care System,' in Robert Evans and G.L. Stoddart, eds., *Medicare at Maturity* (Calgary: University of Calgary Press, 1986). Tuohy, 'Health Care in Canada,' in William M. Chandler and Christian W. Zollner, eds., *Challenges to Federalism: Policy Making in Canada and the Federal Republic of Germany* (Kingston: Institute of Intergovernmental Relations, 1989). Tuohy, *Policy and Politics in Canada: Institutionalized Ambivalence* (Philadelphia: Temple University Press, 1992). Tuohy, ' Social Policy: Two Worlds,' in Michael Atkinson, ed., *Governing Canada: Institutions and Public Policy* (Toronto: Harcourt Brace Jovanovich, 1993). Tuohy, 'Medicine and the State in Canada: The Extra-Billing Issue in Perspective,' *Canadian Journal of Political Science* 21/2 (1988).

9 Miriam Smith, 'Retrenching the Sacred Trust: Medicare and Canadian Federalism,' in Francois Rocher and Miriam Smith, eds., *New Trends in Canadian Federalism* (Peterborough: Broadview, 1995), 320.

10 Tuohy, *Accidental Logics*, 23.

11 Ibid., 204.

12 Ibid., 217 20.

13 See Paul Barker, 'Is the Canada Health Act Important?' paper presented at the Annual Meeting of the Canadian Political Science Association, University of Ottawa, June 1998.

14 See Malcolm H. Taylor, Michael Stevenson, and A. Paul Williams, *Medical Perspectives on Canadian Medicare: Attitudes of Canadian Physicians to Policies*

and Problems of the Medical Care Insurance Program (Toronto: York University, Institute for Behavioural Research, 1984).

15 In the congressional system, the answer to this question is straightforward and relates directly to political institutional logic. But in Canada, there are relatively few institutional constraints or 'veto points.' See Antonia Maioni, *Parting at the Crossroads: The Emergence of Health Insurance in the United States and Canada* (Princeton: Princeton University Press, 1998), 21. In contradistinction, the parliamentary system enables major political transformation with limited legislative resistance.

16 See Canada, Department of Finance, *Budget 1999. Building Today for a Better Tomorrow: Federal Financial Support for the Provinces and Territories*, February 1999, 15.

17 Paul Adams, 'It's an Election Budget,' *Globe and Mail*, 29 February 2000. See also Canada, Department of Finance, *Transfer Payments to Provinces*, February 2001, www.fin.gc.ca/FEDPROV/chse.html (site visited on 3 June 2001).

18 Canada, Department of Finance, *Transfer Payments to Provinces* February 2001, www.fin.gc.ca/FEDPROV/chse.html (site visited on 3 June 2001).

19 David Naylor, 'Health Care in Canada: Incrementalism under Fiscal Duress,' *Health Affairs*, May/June 1999, 23.

20 Canadian Institute for Health Information (CIHI) and Statistics Canada, *Health Care in Canada 2001*, 9 (www.cihi.ca).

21 Ibid., 11.

22 Pat Armstrong and Hugh Armstrong, *Wasting Away: The Undermining of Canadian Health Care* (Toronto: Oxford University Press, 1996). Armstrong and Armstrong, *Universal Health Care: What the United States Can Learn from the Canadian Experience* (New York: New Press, 1998).

23 See Angus Reid Group, 'Public Policy Focus: Canadians' Perspectives on Their Health Care System,' *Angus Reid Report*, January/February 1997. See also Naylor, *Health Care in Canada*, 23.

24 See CIHI and Statistics Canada, *Health Care in Canada 2001*, 23.

25 Tuohy, *Accidental Logics*.

26 Ibid., 34.

27 Ibid.

28 Ibid., 95.

29 The provinces refused to formally participate in the national dialogue of the forum, although the composition of the commission was regionally balanced. See Carolyn Tuohy, *Accidental Logics*, 95.

30 Canada, National Forum on Health, *Canada Health Action: Building on the*

Legacy. The Final Report of the National Forum on Health, 1 (1997), 20. Tuohy, *Accidental Logics,* 96.

31 Ibid., 220.
32 Ibid., 219.
33 Canada, Health Canada, Policy and Consultation Branch, *National Health Expenditures in Canada, 1975–1996. Fact Sheets,* June 1997, 4, figure 3.
34 Ibid., 5, table 1.
35 See CIHI and Statistics Canada, *Health Care in Canada 2001,* 72.
36 Canada, Department of Finance, *Budget 1999. Building Today for a Better Tomorrow: Federal Financial Support for the Provinces and Territories,* February (1999), 15.
37 Ibid., 14.
38 Canada, Department of Finance, *Transfer Payments to Provinces,* February 2001 www. fin.gc.ca/FEDPROV/chse.html (site visited on 3 June 2001).
39 Ibid.
40 Aaron Wildavsky and Naomi Caiden, *The New Politics of the Budgetary Process* (New York: Longman, 1997), 71.
41 Ibid.
42 See Daniel Bell, *The Coming of Post-Industrial Society* (New York: Basic Books, 1973).
43 See Maioni, *Parting at the Crossroads.*
44 Wildavsky and Caiden, *The New Politics of the Budgetary Process,* 96.
45 Keynes' counter-cyclical economic doctrine challenged much of the prevailing wisdom on economic management. According to Keynes, budget deficits are sometimes necessary and desirable to stimulate the economy. This means that during the 'bad times' of economic downturns governments do not have to increase taxes and cut spending. Rather, as Wildavsky explains, 'politicians could finally justify doing what they had long desired to do, namely, do something (spend) to help people (and, in turn, help the economy) in a time of crisis' (ibid., 70). Conversely, during times of growth and relative abundance, that is, 'good times,' spending should be limited and taxation increased to keep the economy from overheating. Put in terms of political appearance, "times are good so we should do less because citizens can afford to pay (their real income is rising) and they won't notice' (ibid.). Not surprisingly, it was difficult for governments to curtail spending for entitlement programs during 'good times.'
46 Tuohy, 'Medicine and the State in Canada.'
47 Canada, Health Canada, *National Health Expenditures in Canada 1975–1996,* Policy and Consultation Branch, June 1997. See also CIHI and Statistics

Canada, *Health Care in Canada: A First Annual Report* (2000), 17, www.cihi.ca.

48 Jane Coutts, 'Cutbacks Are Over, Health Data Suggest,' *Globe and Mail*, 21 August 1997.

49 Ibid.

50 In 2001 the CIHI reported a projected increase in proportion of public expenditure for health care. See CIHI and Statistics Canada, *Health Care in Canada 2001*, 72.

51 Ibid.

52 See Robert J. Blendon, Karen Donelan, and Katherine Binns, *Commonwealth Fund International Health Policy Survey: Summary of Key Findings*, mimeo, September 1998. See also Karen Donelan, Robert J. Blendon, Cathy Schoen, Karen Davis, and Katherine Binns, 'The Cost of Health System Change: Public Discontent in Five Nations,' *Health Affairs* 18/3 (1999), 206–16.

53 David Naylor, 'Health Care in Canada: Incrementalism under Fiscal Duress.' *Health Affairs*, May/June 1999, 23.

54 Cited in ibid., 23.

55 Ibid.

56 See, for example, Paul Pierson. *Dismantling the Welfare State? Reagan, Thatcher and the Politics of Retrenchment* (Cambridge: Cambridge University Press, 1994). Also, Ramesh Mishra, *The Welfare State in Crisis: Social Thought and Social Change* (Sussex: Wheatsheaf Books, 1984).

57 Paul Barker, 'The Development of Major Shared-Cost Programmes in Canada,' in R.D. Olling and M.W. Westmacott, eds., *Perspectives on Canadian Federalism* (Scarborough, Ont.: Prentice-Hall, 1988), 205.

58 Ibid., 210.

59 Thomas Courchene, *Social Canada in the Millennium: Reform Imperatives and Restructuring Principles* (Toronto: C.D. Howe Institute, 1994), 113.

60 From J. Stefan Dupré, 'Comment: The Promise of Procurement Federalism,' in Keith Banting, Douglas Brown, and Thomas Courchene, eds., *The Future of Fiscal Federalism* (Kingston: Queen's University School of Policy Studies, 1994), 250.

61 Miriam Smith, 'Retrenching the Sacred Trust: Medicare and Canadian Federalism,' in François Rocher and Miriam Smith, eds., *New Trends in Canadian Federalism* (Peterborough: Broadview Press, 1995), 328.

62 Courchene, *Social Canada in the Millennium*, 181.

63 Smith, '*Retrenching the Sacred Trust*,' 328.

64 The strength of the medical profession in the health arena and the absence of a similarly powerful interest group in the field of income maintenance

might account for the sharp difference between the two areas of social spending. See Tuohy, 'Social Policy: Two Worlds,' 292–3.

65 When Esping-Andersen's 'welfare worlds' model is applied to Canada, it is evident that health care fits into the social democratic world, and income maintenance programs fit into the liberal world. See Gregg M. Olsen, 'Locating the Canadian Welfare State: Family Policy and Health Care in Canada, Sweden and the United States,' *Canadian Journal of Sociology* 19/1 (1994), 1–20.

66 See Robert G. Evans, Morris L. Barer, and Theodore R. Marmor, *Why Are Some People Healthy and Others Not? Determinants of Health of Populations* (New York: De Gruyter, 1994).

67 Federal, Provincial, and Territorial Advisory Committee on Population Health, *Strategies for Population Health: Investing in the Health of Canadians*, prepared for the meeting of the Ministers of Health, Halifax, Nova Scotia, 14–15 September 1994.

68 Canada, Canadian Intergovernmental Conference Secretariat, News Release. First Ministers' Meeting, Ottawa, Ontario, 11 September 2000. *First Ministers' Meeting: Communiqué on Health*, www.scics.gc.ca/info00/800038004_e.html (site visited on 3 June 2001).

6 Medicine, Health, and Inequality

1 Carolyn Hughes Tuohy, *Accidental Logics: The Dynamics of Change in the Health Care Arena in the United States, Britain, and Canada* (New York: Oxford University Press, 1999), 203–4.

2 See Pat Armstrong and Hugh Armstrong, *Wasting Away: The Undermining of Canadian Health Care* (Toronto: Oxford University Press, 1996); and Patricia O'Reilly, *Health Care Practitioners* (Toronto: University of Toronto Press, 2000).

3 Tuohy, *Accidental Logics*, 12–15.

4 Canadian Institute for Health Information (CIHI) and Statistics Canada, *Health Care in Canada 2001*, 10, www.cihi.ca.

5 Ibid., 10–11.

6 Armstrong and Armstrong, *Wasting Away*, 35–8.

7 CIHI and Statistics Canada, Health Care in Canada: A First Annual Report (2000), 16.

8 Armstrong and Armstrong, *Wasting Away*, 23–4.

9 Ibid., 26.

10 Patricia O'Reilly, *Health Care Practitioners* (Toronto: University of Toronto Press, 2000), 35–6.

11 James Morone, *The Democratic Wish: Popular Participation and the Limits of American Government* (New Haven: Yale University Press, 1990) chapter 7, 285.

12 Carolyn Tuohy, 'Medicine and the State in Canada: The Extra-Billing Issue in Perspective,' *Canadian Journal of Political Science* 21/2 (1988).

13 Ibid.

14 Ibid.

15 Ibid., 278–9.

16 See O'Reilly, *Health Care Practitioners*.

17 See Thomas Courchene, 'ACCESS: A Convention on the Canadian Economic and Social Systems,' in *Assessing Access: Towards a New Social Union. Proceedings of the Symposium on the Courchene Proposal* (Kingston: Institute of Intergovernmental Relations, Queen's University, 1997); Steven Kennett, *Securing the Social Union: A Commentary on the Decentralized Approach* Kingston: Institute of Intergovernmental Relations, Queen's University, 1998), Research Paper no. 34.

18 Harvey Lazar, 'The Federal Role in a New Social Union: Ottawa at a Crossroads,' in Harvey Lazar, ed., *Canada: The State of the Federation. Non-Constitutional Renewal* (Kingston: Institute for Intergovernmental Relations, Queen's University, 1997), 126.

19 See Armstrong and Armstrong, *Wasting Away,* 21.

20 Ibid., 75–7.

21 Janet Lum, 'Paying the Piper: The Regulated Health Professions Act, Health Restructuring and the Costs to Women,' paper presented to the Annual Meeting of the Canadian Political Science Association, University of Ottawa, June 1998, 3.

22 Ibid., 11–12.

23 O'Reilly, *Health Care Practitioners,* 21.

24 Lum, 'Paying the Piper,' 20.

25 Ibid., 5.

26 Malcolm Taylor, H. Michael Stevenson, and A. Paul Williams, *Medical Perspectives on Canadian Medicare: Attitudes of Canadian Physicians to Policies and Problems of the Medical Care Insurance Program* (Toronto: York University, Institute for Behavioural Research, 1984), 58.

27 Ian Harvey, 'Philosophical Perspectives on Priority Setting,' in Joanna Coast, J. Donovan, and S. Frankel, eds., *Priority Setting: The Health Care Debate* (Wiley, 1996).

28 Michael Hayes and Sholom Glouberman, 'Population Health, Sustainable Development and Policy Future,' Canadian Policy Research Networks Discussion Paper, H/01, September 1999, 6.

29 Tee L. Guidotti, '"Why Are Some People Healthy and Others Not?" A Critique of the Population Health Model,' *Annals RCPSC* (Royal College of Physicians and Surgeons of Canada) 30/4, June 1997, 204.

30 For a comprehensive examination of the population health model, see Robert G. Evans, Morris L. Barer, and Theodore R. Marmor, eds., *Why Are Some People Healthy and Others Not? Determinants of Health of Populations* (New York: De Gruyter, 1994); see also Federal, Provincial, and Territorial Advisory Committee on Population Health, *Strategies for Population Health: Investing in the Health of Canadians*. Prepared for the meeting of the Ministers of Health, Halifax, Nova Scotia, 14–15 September 1994.

31 Federal, Provincial, and Territorial Advisory Committee on Population Health, *Strategies for Population Health: Investing in the Health of Canadians*.

32 Evans, 'Introduction' to *Why Are Some People Healthy?* 5.

33 Ibid., 7.

34 World Health Organization (WHO), *The World Health Report, 1999: Making a Difference* (Geneva: World Health Organization, 1999), 16.

35 Ibid., 16–17.

36 Ibid., 33. These statements are meant to indicate broad agreement with the approach of the 'new universalism,' and not an endorsement of the specifics of the WHO approach.

37 See Evans, Barer, and Marmor, *Why Are Some People Healthy?*

38 See '75 Per Cent of Canadians in Favour of Health Care User Fees, Poll Finds,' *National Post*, 12 January 2000; Jeff Heinrich, 'Quebec Poll Finds Support for Private Health Care,' *National Post*, 29 December 1999.

7 Citizenship Entitlement, Community: Evaluation Community Governance Structures

1 See Jonathan Lomas, John Woods, and Gerry Veenstra, 'Devolving Authority for Health Care in Canada's Provinces: An Introduction to the Issues,' *CMAJ* 156/3 (1997), 371–7. Lomas, Woods, and Veenstra, 'Devolving Authority for Health Care in Canada's Provinces. Backgrounds, Resources, and Activities of Board Members,' *CMAJ* 156/4 (1997). Lomas, Woods, and Veenstra, 'Devolving Authority for Health Care in Canada's Provinces. Motivations, Attitudes and Approaches of Board Members,' *CMAJ*,156/5 (1997). Lomas, Woods, and Veenstra, 'Devolving Authority for Health Care in Canada's Provinces. Emerging Issues and Prospects,' *CMAJ* 156/6 (1997). Jonathan Lomas and Michael Rachlis, 'Moving Rocks: Block Funding in PEI as an Incentive for Cross-Sectoral Reallocations among Human Services,' *Canadian Public Administration* 39/4 (1996).

2 Pat Armstrong and Hugh Armstrong, *Wasting Away: The Undermining of Canadian Health Care* (Toronto: Oxford University Press, 1996), 13.

3 Gosta Esping-Andersen, 'Citizenship and Socialism: De-Commodification and Solidarity in the Welfare State,' in Martin Rein and Lee Rainwater, eds., *Stagnation and Renewal in Social Policy* (New York: Sharpe, 1987).

4 Carolyn Hughes Tuohy, 'Conflict and Accommodation in the Canadian Health Care System,' in Robert Evans and G.L. Stoddart, eds., *Medicare at Maturity* (Calgary: University of Calgary Press, 1986); Tuohy, 'Health Care in Canada,' in William M. Chandler and Christian W. Zollner, eds., *Challenges to Federalism: Policy-Making in Canada and the Federal Republic of Germany* (Kingston: Institute of Intergovernmental Relations, 1989); Tuohy, *Policy and Politics in Canada: Institutionalized Ambivalence* (Philadelphia: Temple University Press, 1992).

5 Joanna Coast, 'Core Services: Pluralistic Bargaining in New Zealand,' in J. Coast, J. Donovan, and S. Frankel, eds., *Priority Setting: The Health Care Debate* (New York: Wiley, 1996); Lomas and Rachlis, 'Moving Rocks,' 586.

6 On 1 February 1994, the Oregon Plan took effect; 565 out of the 696 treatment/condition pairs were funded. Joanna Coast, 'The Oregon Plan: Technical Priority Setting in the USA,' in J. Coast, J. Donovan, and S. Frankel, eds., *Priority Setting: The Health Care Debate* (New York: Wiley, 1996), 47.

7 Thomas Courchene, 'ACCESS: A Convention on the Canadian Economic and Social Systems,' In *Assessing ACCESS: Proceedings of the Symposium on the Courchene Proposal* (Kingston: Queen's University, Institute of Intergovernmental Relations, 1997), 81.

8 Nova Scotia, *The Report of the Nova Scotia Royal Commission on Health Care: Towards a New Strategy* (Halifax: December 1989).

9 Nova Scotia, The Minister's Action Committee on Health System Reform, *Nova Scotia's Blueprint for Health System Reform* (Halifax: Department of Health, 1994), 17.

10 Ibid., 26.

11 Nova Scotia, The Minister's Action Committee on Health System Reform, *From Blueprint to Building: Renovating Nova Scotia's Health System* (Halifax: Department of Health, 1995), 6.

12 Ibid., 7.

13 The initial process of regionalization in Nova Scotia created four Regional Health Boards, with a total of 67 members (all appointed by government – some salaried, some on a volunteer basis), and 30 Community Health Boards with a total of approximately 420 members. Nova Scotia: Department of Health, *Health Care Update – Regionalization* (December 1997), 10.

14 Ibid.

15 These are the Queen Elizabeth the II Health Sciences Centre in Halifax and the Cape Breton Regional Hospital.
16 The IWK-Grace and the Nova Scotia Hospital.
17 See Nova Scotia, Department of Health, *Future Direction of the Health Care System: Establishing District Health Authorities*, 1 November 1999.
18 For a detailed account of implementation of health districts in Saskatchewan, see HealNet: Health Services Utilization and Research Commission, *Regionalization at Age Five: Views of Saskatchewan Health Care Decision-Makers*, December 1997.
19 Confidential interview, October 1998.
20 James Morone, *The Democratic Wish: Popular Participation and the Limits of American Government* (New Haven: Yale University Press, 1990), 285.
21 In 1996 AFDC was replaced with a block grant. See Gary Bryner, *Politics and Public Morality: The Great American Welfare Reform Debate* (New York: Norton, 1998).
22 Michael Brannigan, 'Oregon's Experiment,' in David Seedhouse, ed., *Reforming Health Care: The Philosophy and Practice of International Health Reform* (New York: Wiley, 1995), 27.
23 David Eddy, 'Clinical Decision-Making: From Theory to Practice. What's Going on in Oregon?' *JAMA* 266/3 (1991), 419.
24 Harvey D. Klevit et al., 'Prioritization of Health Care Services: A Progress Report of the Oregon Health Services Commission,' *Archives of Internal Medicine* 151/5 (1991), 913.
25 Eddy, 'Clinical Decision-Making,' 419.
26 Brannigan, 'Oregon's Experiment,' 29.
27 Theodore Ganiats and Robert Kaplan, 'Priority Setting: The Oregon Example,' in F. Schwartz, H. Glennerster, and R. Saltman, eds., *Fixing Health Budgets: Experience from Europe and North America* (New York: Wiley, 1996), 21.
28 Daniel Fox and Howard Leichter, 'Rationing Health Care in Oregon: The New Accountability,' *Health Affairs* 10/2 (1991), 22.
29 Fox and Leichter explain that 'Oregonians, ever mindful of the history of the Oregon Trail and of courageous pioneers, take pride in their innovative social policy. More recently, the *Almanac of American Politics* described Oregon as "a culturally liberal state on many issues, with many young and single voters, and one that is proud of being the first state to ban throwaway bottles and among the first to allow abortions." The popular image that Oregonians have of themselves has been called a "moralistic" political subculture, in which "both the general public and politicians conceive of politics as a public activity centered on some notion of the public

good and properly devoted to the advancement of the public interest"' (ibid., 16). Oregon is exceptional in many respects, but citizen participation or community engagement is a feature of many other state political cultures.

30 Coast, 'The Oregon Plan,' 38.
31 Ibid.
32 Ibid.
33 Ibid.
34 Fox and Leichter, 'Rationing Health Care in Oregon,' 22.
35 Ibid.
36 Ibid.
37 Gail McBride, 'Bush Vetoes Health care Rationing in Oregon,' *BMJ* 305/6851 (1992), 437.
38 Brannigan, 'Oregon's Experiment,' 32.
39 Lomas and Rachlis, 'Moving Rocks,' 586.
40 Nova Scotia, Department of Health, *Future Directions*, 3.
41 This analysis is consistent with proponents of deliberative democracy who explain that free and open communication among the citizenry is an essential component of democratic public-policy making. In general terms, more citizen participation means greater diversity of opinion. By inviting everyone to the discursive forum, politics become less elitist and exclusive and, ultimately, better decisions will result. At the very least, decisions will be more legitimate in that the process through which they were deliberated was open, and dissenting voices were heard.
42 Lawrence Jacobs, Theodore Marmor, and Jonathan Oberlander, 'The Oregon Health Plan and the Political Paradox of Rationing: What Advocates and Critics Have Claimed and What Oregon Did,' *Journal of Health Politics, Policy and Law* 24/1 (1999), 172.
43 Ibid.
44 Ibid.
45 See also John Dryzek, *Discursive Democracy: Politics, Policy and Political Science* (Cambridge: Cambridge University Press, 1994); Amy Bartholomew, 'Democratic Citizenship, Social Rights and the 'Reflexive Continuation' of the Welfare State,' *Studies in Political Economy* 42 (Autumn 1993), 141–56; Lynn Sanders, 'Against Deliberation,' *Political Theory* 25/3 (1997), 347–77.
46 See Jane Mansbridge, 'The Limits of Friendship,' in John Arthur, ed., *Democracy: Theory and Practice* (Belmont: Wadsworth, 1991); and Sanders, 'Against Deliberation.'
47 Jon Elster, 'Three Varieties of Political Theory,' in James Bohman and

William Rehg, eds., *Deliberative Democracy: Essays on Reason and Politics* (Cambridge: MIT Press, 1997), 3.

48 Jean-Jacques Rousseau, 'Letter to M. D'Alembert on the Theatre,' in Allan Bloom, trans., *Politics and the Arts* (New York: Free Press, 1960), 17.

49 Ibid., 25.

50 Carole Pateman, 'A Participatory Theory of Democracy,' in John Arthur, ed., *Democracy: Theory and Practice* (Belmont: Wadsworth, 1991), 118.

51 Mansbridge, 'The Limits of Friendship,' 125.

52 Sanders, 'Against Deliberation.'

53 See Cass Sunstein, 'Beyond the Republican Revival,' *Yale Law Review* 97 (1988), 1539–90; Bruce Ackerman, *Social Justice in the Liberal State* (New Haven: Yale University Press, 1980); and James S. Fishkin, *Democracy and Deliberation* (New Haven: Yale University Press, 1991).

54 Cohen and Rogers argue that differences in social class will serve as barriers to equal opportunities for deliberation. Joshua Cohen and Joel Rogers, *On Democracy* (New York: Penguin, 1983).

55 Lomas, Veenstra, and Woods, 'Devolving Authority for Health Care in Canada's Provinces: Backgrounds, Resources and Activities of Board Members,' *CMAJ* 156 (1997), 513–20.

56 Ibid.

57 Simon Watney, 'Practices of Freedom: "Citizenship" and the Politics of Identity in the Age of AIDS,' in Jonathan Rutherford, ed., *Identity: Community Culture Difference* (New York: New York University Press, 1990).

58 See Halifax Peninsula Community Health Board, *Halifax Peninsula Community Health Plan. Condensed Version of the Issues and Recommendations Sections Only.*

59 See Will Kymlicka and Wayne Norman, 'Return of the Citizen: A Survey of Recent Work on Citizenship Theory,' in Ronald Beiner, ed., *Theorizing Citizenship* (Albany: State University of New York Press, 1995). The authors explain that 'the New Right believes that the model of passive citizenship underestimated the extent to which fulfilling certain obligations is a precondition for being accepted as a full member of society' (287). And 'most people on the left continue to defend the principle that full citizenship requires social rights' (288).

8 Conclusion: Health Care and Universality: Looking Ahead

1 World Health Organization, *Making a Difference* (Geneva: WHO 1999), 33.

2 Ibid.

3 See Michael Hayes and Sholom Glouberman, 'Population Health, Sustainable Development and Policy Future,' Canadian Policy Research Network Discussion paper H/01, September 1999, 21.

References

Ackerman, Bruce. *Social Justice in the Liberal State*. New Haven: Yale University Press, 1980.

Adams, Paul, 'It's an Election Budget.' *Globe and Mail*, 29 February 2000.

Adelson, Naomi. *'Being Alive Well': Health and the Politics of Cree Well-Being*. Toronto: University of Toronto Press, 2000.

Angus Reid Group. 'Public Policy Focus: Canadians' Perspectives on Their Health Care System,' *The Angus Reid Report*, January–February 1997, 31–71.

Appiah, K. Anthony. 'Race, Culture, Identity: Misunderstood Connections.' In K. Anthony Appiah and Amy Gutmann, *Color Conscious: The Political Morality of Race* 30–105. Princeton: Princeton University Press, 1996.

Armstrong, Pat. 'Unravelling the Safety Net: Transformations in Health Care and Their Impact on Women.' In Janine Brodie ed., *Women and Canadian Public Policy*, 129–49. Toronto: Harcourt Brace, 1996.

Armstrong, Pat, and Hugh Armstrong. *Universal Health Care: What the United States Can Learn from the Canadian Experience*. New York: The New Press, 1998.

– *Wasting Away: The Undermining of Canadian Health Care*. Toronto: Oxford University Press, 1996.

Barbalet, J.M. *Citizenship: Rights Struggle and Class Inequality*. Minneapolis: University of Minnesota Press, 1988.

Barker, Paul. 'Is the Canada Health Act Important?' Paper presented at the Annual Meeting of the Canadian Political Science Association, University of Ottawa, June 1998.

– 'The Development of Major Shared-Cost Programmes in Canada.' In R.D. Olling and M.W. Westmacott eds., *Perspectives on Canadian Federalism*, 195–219. Scarborough, Ont. Prentice-Hall Canada, 1988.

Bartholomew, Amy. 'Democratic Citizenship, Social Rights and the 'Reflexive Continuation' of the Welfare State,' *Studies in Political Economy* 42 (Autumn 1993), 141–56.

Bazowski, Raymond. 'Canadian Political Thought.' In James Bickerton and Alain Gagnon eds., *Canadian Politics*, 93–109. Peterborough: Broadview Press, 1995.

Beiner, Ronald. *Philosophy in a Time of Lost Spirit.* Toronto: University of Toronto Press, 1997.

– ed., *Theorizing Citizenship.* Albany: State University of New York Press, 1995.

– *What's the Matter with Liberalism?* (Berkeley and Los Angeles: University of California Press, 1992.

Bell, Daniel. *The Coming of Post-Industrial Society.* New York: Basic Books, 1973.

Blendon, Robert J., Karen Donelan, and Katherine Binns. *Commonwealth Fund International Health Policy Survey: Summary of Key Findings.* Mimeo, September 1998.

Boase, Joan Price. *Shifting Sands: Government-Group Relations in the Health Care Sector.* Montreal and Kingston: McGill-Queen's University Press, 1994.

Brannigan, Michael. 'Oregon's Experiment.' In David Seedhouse ed., *Reforming Health Care: The Philosophy and Practice of International Health Reform*, chapter 2. New York: John Wiley and Sons Ltd., 1995.

Bryner, Gary. *Politics and Public Morality: The Great American Welfare Reform Debate.* New York: W.W. Norton, 1998.

Caiden, Naomi. 'Public Budgeting amidst Uncertainty and Instability.' In Jay Shafritz and Albert Hyde, eds., *Classics of Public Administration*, 485–96. 3rd ed. Pacific Grove, Calif.: Brooks/Cole, 1992.

– 'Negative Financial Management: A Backward Look at Fiscal Stress.' In Charles Levine and Irene Rubin eds., *Fiscal Stress and Public Policy*, 135–58. London: Sage, 1980.

Cameron v Nova Scotia (A.G.) (1997), 163 N.S.R. (2d) 391, 487 A.P.R. 391 (S.C.)

Canada, Canadian Intergovernmental Conference Secretariat. News Release. First Ministers' Meeting, Ottawa, Ontario, 11 Sept. 2000. *First Ministers' Meeting: Communiqué on Health.* www.scics.gc.ca/info00/800038004_e.html (site visited on 3 June 2001.

Canada, Department of Finance, *Transfer Payments to Provinces.* Feb. 2001. www.fin.gc.ca/FEDPROV/chse.html (site visited on 3 June 2001).

– *Budget 1999. Building Today for a Better Tomorrow: Federal Financial Support for the Provinces and Territories.* February 1999.

Canada, Health Canada: *HIV Testing and Pregnancy: Medical and Legal Parameters of the Policy Debate.* 1999.

– Speaking notes for the Honourable Alan Rock, Minister of Health at the 130th Annual Meeting of the Canadian Medical Association, Victoria, BC, 20 August 1997.

– Policy and Consultation Branch. *National Health Expenditures in Canada 1975– 1996. Fact Sheets*. June 1997.

Canadian Institute for Health Information (CIHI) and Statistics Canada. *Health Care in Canada 2001*. www.cihi.ca.

– *Health Care in Canada: A First Annual Report* (2000). www.cihi.ca.

Canada, National Forum on Health, *Canada Health Action: Building on the Legacy. The Final Report of the National Forum on Health*. Vol. 1 (1997).

– *Canada Health Action: Building on the Legacy*. Synthesis Reports and Issues Papers, vol. 2 (1997).

Canadian Public Health Association. *Health Impacts of Social and Economic Conditions: Implications for Public Policy*. CPHA Board of Directors Discussion Paper, Ottawa, March 1997.

Cernetig, Miro. 'Alberta Doctors Attack Cuts in Health Care,' *Globe and Mail*, 17 November 1995.

Charles, Cathy, Jonathan Lomas, and Mita Giacomini. 'Medical Necessity in Canadian Health Policy: Four Meanings and ... a Funeral?' *Milbank Quarterly* 75/3 (September 1997).

Coast, Joanna. 'Core Services: Pluralistic Bargaining in New Zealand.' In J. Coast, J. Donovan, and S. Frankel, eds., *Priority Setting: The Health Care Debate*, 65–82. New York: Wiley, 1996.

– 'The Oregon Plan: Technical Priority Setting in the USA.' In J. Coast, J. Donovan, and S. Frankel eds., *Priority Setting: The Health Care Debate*, New York: Wiley, 1996.

Cohen, Joshua, and Joel Rogers. *On Democracy*. New York: Penguin, 1983.

Courchene, Thomas. 'ACCESS: A Convention on the Canadian Economic and Social Systems,' Working paper prepared for the Ministry of Intergovernmental Affairs, Government of Ontario. Reprinted in *Assessing Access: Towards a New Social Union. Proceedings of the Symposium on the Courchene Proposal*. Kingston: Institute of Intergovernmental Relations, Queen's University, 1996.

– *Social Canada in the Millennium: Reform Imperatives and Restructuring Principles*. Toronto: C.D. Howe Institute, 1994.

Coutts, Jane. 'Cutbacks Are Over, Health Data Suggest.' *Globe and Mail*, 21 August 1997.

– 'Physicians Fear Health Funds Draining from Medical Care.' *Globe and Mail*, 20 August 1997.

Cunningham, William E., R.M. Anderson, M.H. Katrz, M.D. Stein, B.J. Turner,

S. Crystal, S. Zierler, K. Kuromiya, S.C. Morton, P. St. Clair, S.A. Bozzette, and M.F. Shapiro. 'The Impact of Competing Subsistence Needs and Barriers on Access to Medical Care for Persons with Human Immunodeficiency Virus Receiving Care in the United States.' *Medical Care* 37/12 (December 1999).

Dahrendorf, Ralf. 'The Changing Quality of Citizenship.' In Bart van Steenbergen, ed., *The Condition of Citizenship*, 10–19. London: Sage, 1994.

– *The Modern Social Conflict: An Essay on the Politics of Liberty.* New York: Weidenfeld and Nicolson, 1988.

Deber, Raisa. 'The Use and Misuse of Economics.' In Margaret A. Somerville, ed., *Do We Care? Renewing Canada's Commitment to Health*, 53–68. Montreal: McGill-Queen's University Press, 1999.

DeCoster, Carolyn, and Marni Brownell. 'Private Health Care in Canada: Savior or Siren?' *Public Health Reports* 112 (July–August 1997).

Dickinson, Harley. 'The Struggle for State Health Insurance: Reconsidering the Role of Saskatchewan Farmers.' *Studies in Political Economy* 41 (Summer 1993), 133–56.

Doern, G. Bruce, and Glen Toner. *The Politics of Energy: The Development and Implementation of the NEP.* Toronto: Methuen, 1985.

Donelan, Karen, Robert J. Blendon, Cathy Schoen, Karen Davis, and Katherine Binns. 'The Cost of Health System Change: Public Discontent in Five Nations.' *Health Affairs* 18/3 (1999), 206–16.

Downie, J., and T. Caulfield, eds. *Canadian Health Law and Policy.* Toronto: Butterworth, 1999.

Dryzek, John. *Discursive Democracy: Politics, Policy and Political Science.* Cambridge: Cambridge University Press, 1994.

Dupré, J. Stefan. 'Comment: The Promise of Procurement Federalism.' In Keith Banting, Douglas Brown, and Thomas Courchene, eds., *The Future of Fiscal Federalism*, 249–59. Kingston: Queen's University School of Policy Studies, 1994.

– 'Reflections on the Workability of Executive Federalism.' In R.D. Olling and M.W. Westmacott, eds., *Perspectives on Canadian Federalism*. Scarborough, Ont.: Prentice Hall, 1988. 223–56.

Dworkin, Ronald. *Life's Dominion.* New York: Vintage Books, 1994.

– *Foundations of Liberal Equality,* Tanner Lectures on Human Values XI. Salt Lake City: University of Utah Press, 1990.

– *Taking Rights Seriously.* London: Duckworth, 1978.

Dyck, Arthur J. *Rethinking Rights and Responsibilities: The Moral Bonds of Community.* Cleveland: Pilgrim Press, 1994.

Eddy, David M. 'Clinical Decision-Making: From Theory to Practice. What's Going on in Oregon?' *JAMA* 266/3 (1991), 417–20.

Eldridge v *British Columbia (Attorney General)*, [1997] 3 S.C.R. 624.

Elster, Jon. 'The Market and the Forum: Three Varieites of Political Theory.' In James Bohman and William Rehg, eds., *Deliberative Democracy: Essays on Reason and Politics*, 3–33. Cambridge: MIT Press, 1997.

Esping-Andersen, Gosta. *The Three Worlds of Welfare Capitalism*. Princeton: Princeton University Press, 1990.

– 'Citizenship and Socialism: De-Commodification and Solidarity in the Welfare State.' In Martin Rein and Lee Rainwater, eds., *Stagnation and Renewal in Social Policy*. New York: Sharpe, 1987.

– *Politics Against Markets: The Social Democratic Road to Power*. Princeton: Princeton University Press, 1985.

– 'Power and Distributional Regimes.' *Politics and Society* 14 (1985) 223–56.

Etzioni, Amitai. *The Limits of Privacy*. New York: Basic Books, 1999.

Evans, Robert G. 'Canada: The Real Issues.' *Journal of Health Politics, Policy and Law* 17/2 (1992), 739–62.

– 'Hang Together or Hang Separately: The Viability of a Universal Health Care System in an Aging Society.' *Canadian Public Policy* 13/2 (1987) 165–80.

Evans, Robert G., Morris L. Barer, and Theodore R. Marmor, eds. *Why Are Some People Healthy and Others Not? Determinants of Health of Populations*. New York: De Gruyter, 1994.

Farmer, Paul. *Infections and Inequalities: The Modern Plagues*. Berkeley and Los Angeles: University of California Press, 1999.

Federal, Provincial, and Territorial Advisory Committee on Population Health. *Strategies for Population Health: Investing in the Health of Canadians*. Prepared for the meeting of the Ministers of Health, Halifax, Nova Scotia, 14–15 September 1994.

Feinberg, Joel. 'The Nature and Value of Rights.' In David Lyons, ed., *Rights*, 78–91. Belmont: Wadsworth, 1979.

Fishkin, James S. *Democracy and Deliberation*. New Haven: Yale University Press, 1991.

Flood, Colleen. 'The Structure and Dynamics of Canada's Health Care System.' In J. Downie and T. Caulfield, eds., *Canadian Health Law and Policy*. Toronto: Butterworth, 1999.

Fox, Daniel M., and Howard M. Leichter. 'Rationing Care in Oregon: The New Accountability.' *Health Affairs*, Summer 1991, 7–27.

Franks, C.E.S. *The Parliament of Canada*. Toronto: University of Toronto Press, 1987.

Friedman, Kathi. *Legitimation of Social Rights and the Western Welfare State*. Chapel Hill: University of North Carolina Press, 1981.

Ganiats, Theodore G., and Robert M. Kaplan. 'Priority Setting: the Oregon

Example.' In F.W. Schwartz, H. Glennerster and Richard B. Saltman, eds., *Fixing Health Budgets: Experience From Europe and North America*. New York: Wiley, 1996.

'Gambling with Medicare,' *Saturday Night*, March 1996, 44–50.

Glendon, Mary Ann. *Rights Talk: The Impoverishment of Political Discourse*. New York: Free Press, 1991.

Goold, Susan. 'Allocating Health Care: Cost-Utility Analysis, Informed Democratic Decision-Making, or the Veil of Ignorance?' *Journal of Health Politics, Policy and Law*, 21/1 (Spring 1996), 69–98.

Graham, Katherine, and Susan Phillips. 'Citizen Engagement: Beyond the Customer Revolution,' *Canadian Public Administration* 40/2 (Summer 1990), 255–73.

Guidotti, Tee L. 'Why are Some People Healthy and Others Not? A Critique of the Population Health Model.' *Annals* RCPSC (Royal College of Physicians and Surgeons of Canada), 30/4 (June 1997), 203–6.

Gutmann, Amy, ed., *Multiculturalism: Examining the Politics of Recognition*. Princeton: Princeton University Press, 1994.

Halifax Peninsula Community Health Board. *Halifax Peninsula Community Health Plan*. Condensed Version of the Issues and Recommendations Sections Only.

Hall, Emmett. *The Royal Commission on Health Services* (Report), Ottawa: R. Duhamel, Queen's Printer, 1964.

Hart, H.L.A. 'Are There Any Natural Rights?' In David Lyons, ed., *Rights*, 14–25. Belmont: Wadsworth, 1979.

Harvey, Ian. 'Philosophical Perspectives on Priority Setting.' In Joanna Coast et al., eds., *Priority Setting: The Health Care Debate*. New York: Wiley, 1996.

Hayes, Michael, and Sholom Glouberman. 'Population Health, Sustainable Development and Policy Future.' Canadian Policy Research Networks Discussion Paper, H/01, September 1999.

HealNet: Health Services Utilization and Research Commission, *Regionalization at Age Five: Views of Saskatchewan Health Care Decision-Makers*, December 1997.

Heeney, Helen. *Life Before Medicare: Canadian Experiences*. Toronto: Ontario Coalition of Senior Citizens Organizations, 1995.

Heinrich, Jeff. 'Quebec Poll Finds Support for Private Health Care,' *National Post*, 29 December 1999.

Hindness, Barry. 'Citizenship and the Modern West.' In Bryan Turner, ed., *Citizenship and Social Theory*. London: Sage, 1993.

Hunter, David J. *Desperately Seeking Solutions: Rationing Health Care*. New York: Longman, 1997.

'Intensive Care: Can Diane Marleau Rescue Her Damaged Reputation as Health Minister?' *Maclean's*, 23 May 1994, 12–15.

Jacobs, Lawrence, Theodore Marmor, and Jonathan Oberlander 'The Oregon Health Plan and the Political Paradox of Rationing: What Advocates and Critics Have Claimed and What Oregon Did.' *Journal of Health Politics, Policy and Law*, 24/1 (February 1999), 161–80.

Kaiser Family Foundation, *Medicaid and the Uninsured*, May 2000, www.kff.org/content/2000/1420 (site visited on 3 June 2001).

Kant, Immanuel. 'Foundations of the Metaphysics of Morals.' In Lewis White Beck, ed., *Kant Selections*. New York: Macmillan, 1988. Originally published in 1785.

Kennett, Stephen. *Securing the Social Union: A Commentary on the Decentralized Approach*. Kingston: Institute of Intergovernmental Relations, Queen's University, Research Paper no. 34.

Kilborn, Peter. 'Trend toward Managed Care Is Unpopular, Surveys Find.' *New York Times*, 28 September 1997.

– 'Workers Getting Greater Freedom in Health Plans.' *New York Times*, 17 August 1997.

King, Desmond. *The New Right: Politics, Markets and Citizenship*. London: Macmillan, 1987.

King, Desmond, and Jeremy Waldron. 'Citizenship, Social Citizenship and the Defence of Welfare Provision.' *British Journal of Political Science* 18 (1988), 415–43.

Klausen, Jytte. 'Social Rights Advocacy and State Building: T.H. Marshall in the Hands of Social Reformers.' *World Politics* 47/2 (Jan. 1995), 244–67.

Klevit, Harvey D., Alan Bates, Tina Castanares, Paul Kirk, Paige Sipes-Metzler, and Richard Wopat. 'Prioritization of Health Care Services: A Progress Report of the Oregon Health Services Commission,' 912–16. *Archives of Internal Medicine* 151/5 (1991).

Kouri, Denise, Jackie Dutchak, and Steven Lewis. *Regionalization at Age Five: Views of Saskatchewan Health Care Decision-Makers*. HealNet Regional Health Planning, December 1997.

– *Regionalization at Age Five: Views of Saskatchewan Health Care Decision-Makers Supplement: Frequency Distributions*. HealNet Regional Health Planning, December 1997.

Kronick, Richard, and Todd Gilmer. 'Explaining the Decline in Health Insurance Coverage, 1979–1995.' *Health Affairs* 18/2 (1999), 30–47.

Kunst, Anton, and Johan Mackenbach. *Measuring Socioeconomic Inequalities in Health*. Copenhagen: World Health Organization, 1995.

Kymlicka, Will. *Multicultural Citizenship: A Liberal Theory of Minority Rights.* Oxford: Oxford University Press, 1996.

– *Liberalism, Community and Culture.* Oxford: Clarendon Press, 1989.

Kymlicka, Will, and Wayne Norman. *Citizenship in Diverse Societies.* Oxford: Oxford University Press, 2000.

– 'Return of the Citizen: A Survey of Recent Work on Citizenship Theory.' In Ronald Beiner, ed., *Theorizing Citizenship.* Albany: SUNY Press, 1995.

Langlois, Kathy. 'A Saskatchewan Vision for Health: Who Really Makes the Decisions?' In Robin Ford and David Zussman, eds., *Alternative Service Delivery: Sharing Governance in Canada*, 173–84. Toronto: IPAC, 1997.

Lasswell, Harold D. *Politics, Who Gets What, When, How.* New York: Peter Smith, 1950. First published in 1936.

Lazar, Harvey. 'The Federal Role in a New Social Union: Ottawa at a Cross-roads.' In Harvey Lazar, ed., *Canada: The State of the Federation: Non-Constitutional Renewal*, 105–36. Kingston: Institute for Intergovernmental Relations, Queen's University, 1997.

Levine, Charles. 'Organizational Decline and Cutback Management.' In Jay Shafritz and Albert Hyde, eds., *Classics of Public Administration.* Belmont: Wadsworth, 1992. Essay originally published in 1978.

Lindemann Nelson, James. 'Publicity and Pricelessness: Grassroots Decision-Making and Justice in Rationing.' *Journal of Medicine and Philosophy* 19 (1994), 333–42.

Lipsky, Michael. *Street-Level Bureaucracy: Dilemmas of the Individual in Public Services.* Russell Sage Foundation, 1980.

Lomas, Jonathan, and Michael Rachlis. 'Moving Rocks: Block Funding in PEI as an Incentive for Cross-Sectoral Reallocations among Human Services.' *Canadian Public Administration* 39/4, 581–600.

Lomas, Jonathan, John Woods, and Gerry Veenstra. 'Devolving Authority for Health Care in Canada's Provinces: An Introduction to the Issues.' *CMAJ*, 156/3 (1997), 371–7.

– 'Devolving Authority for Health Care in Canada's Provinces: Backgrounds, Resources and Activities of Board Members.' *CMAJ* 156/4 (1997), 513–20.

– 'Devolving Authority for Health Care in Canada's Provinces. Motivations, Attitudes and Approaches of Board Members.' *CMAJ* 156/5 (1997), 669–76.

– 'Devolving Authority for Health Care in Canada's Provinces. 4. Emerging Issues and Prospects.' *CMAJ* 156/6 (1997), 817–23.

Lum, Janet. 'Paying the Piper: The Regulated Health Professions Act, Health Restructuring and the Costs to Women.' Paper presented to the Annual Meeting of the Canadian Political Science Association, University of Ottawa, June 1998.

Macpherson, C.B. *The Political Theory of Possessive Individualism*. Oxford: Oxford University Press, 1962.

Madore, Odette. *The Canada Health Act: Overview and Options*. Ottawa: Economics Division, Research Branch, Library of Parliament, 1995.

Maioni, Antonia. *Parting at the Crossroads: The Emergence of Health Insurance in the United States and Canada*. Princeton: Princeton University Press, 1998.

– 'Nothing Succeeds Like the Right Kind of Failure.' *Journal of Health Politics, Policy and Law* 20/1 (Spring 1995), 5–30.

Mansbridge, Jane. 'The Limits of Friendship.' In John Arthur, ed., *Democracy: Theory and Practice*, 121–32. Belmont: Wadsworth, 1991.

Marmor, Theodore. *The Politics of Medicare*. New York: de Gruyter, 2000.

– *The Politics of Medicare*. New York: de Gruyter, 1973.

Marshall, T.H. *Class, Citizenship and Social Development*. New York: Doubleday, 1964.

Maslove, Allan. *National Goals and the Federal Role in Health Care*. Canada: National Forum on Health, November, 1995.

– 'Time to Fold or Up the Ante: The Federal Role in Health Care.' John F. Graham Memorial Lecture, Dalhousie University, 9 March 1995.

– 'A Theory of Human Motivation.' In Jay Shafritz and Albert Hyde, eds., *Classics of Public Administration*. 3rd ed. Pacific Grove, CA: Brooks/Cole, 1992. Originally published in 1943.

Maslove, Allan, and Kevin Moore. 'From Red Books to Blue Books: Repairing Ottawa's Fiscal House.' In Gene Swimmer, ed., *How Ottawa Spends 1997–98. Seeing Red: A Liberal Report Card*, 23–49. Ottawa: Carleton University Press, 1997.

Maxwell, Judith. 'Social Dimensions of Economic Growth.' Eric J. Hanson Memorial Lecture, University of Alberta, 25 January 1996.

Mead, Lawrence. 'Citizenship and Social Policy: T.H. Marshall and Poverty.' *Social Philosophy and Policy* 14/2 (1997), 197–230.

Miller, Tracey E. 'Managed Care Regulation in the Laboratory of the States.' *JAMA* 278, 1 October 1997.

Minkler, Meredith, ed. *Community Organizing and Community Building for Health*. New Brunswick, NJ: Rutgers University Press, 1997.

Mishra, Ramesh. *The Welfare State in Crisis: Social Thought and Social Change*. Sussex: Wheatsheaf Books, 1984.

Morone, James. *The Democratic Wish: Popular Participation and the Limits of American Government*. New Haven: Yale University Press, 1990.

Naylor, David. 'Evidence-Based Health Care: A Reality Check.' Amyot Lecture delivered at Health Canada, Tunney's Pasture, Ottawa, Ontario, 18 Oct. 2000 www.hc-sc.gc.ca/english/amyot2000_5.htm.

- 'Health Care in Canada: Incrementalism under Fiscal Duress.' *Health Affairs*, May/June 1999, 9–26.
- '*Private Practice, Public Payment: Canadian Medicine and the Politics of Health Insurance*. Montreal: McGill-Queen's University Press, 1986.

Nestman, Lawrence J. 'Federal and Provincial Roles in Canadian Health Care Budgets.' In F.W. Schwartz, H. Glennerster, and R.B. Saltman, eds., *Fixing Health Budgets: Experience from Europe and North America*. New York: Wiley, 1996.

Nova Scotia. *The Report of the Nova Scotia Royal Commission on Health Care: Towards a New Strategy*. Halifax: December 1999.
- Department of Health. *Future Direction of the Health Care System: Establishing District Health Authorities*. November 1999.
- Department of Health. *Health Care Update – Regionalization*. Advance printing December 1997.
- Department of Health. *From Blueprint to Building: Renovating Nova Scotia's Health System*. 1995.
- The Minister's Action Committee on Health System Reform *Nova Scotia's Blueprint for Health System Reform*. 1994.

Nova Scotia Medical Services Insurance. *Physicians' Bulletin*, 7 and 21 February 1997.

Nozick, Robert. *Anarchy, State, and Utopia*. Oxford: Basil Blackwell, 1974.

OECD. *Internal Markets in the Making: Health Systems in Canada, Iceland, and the United Kingdom*. Paris: OECD, 1995.

Olsen, Gregg M. 'Locating the Canadian Welfare State: Family Policy and Health Care in Canada, Sweden and the United States.' *Canadian Journal of Sociology* 19/1 (1994), 1–20.

O'Reilly, Patricia. *Health Care Practitioners*. Toronto: University of Toronto Press, 2000.

Paine, Thomas. 'Agrarian Justice.' In Philip S. Foner, ed., *The Complete Writings of Thomas Paine*. New York: The Citadel Press, 1945. Originally published in 1796.

Pan-American Health Organization (PAHO) / World Health Organization, Division of Health Systems and Services Development. *Series: I. Decentralization, Health Systems and Sectoral Reform Processes. Final Report*. Valdivia, Chile, 17–20 March 1997.

Pan-American Health Organization / Inter-American Development Bank. Caribbean Group for Cooperation in Economic Development. *Caribbean Regional Health Study*. May 1996.

PAHO. *Community Participation in Health and Development in the Americas*. Pan

American Health Organization. Scientific Publications, no. 473. December 1984.

Pal, Leslie. *Interests of State: The Politics of Language, Multiculturalism and Feminism in Canada*. Montreal: McGill-Queen's University Press, 1993.

Parker, Julie. *Social Policy and Citizenship*. London: Macmillan, 1975.

Pateman, Carole. 'A Participatory Theory of Democracy.' In John Arthur, ed., *Democracy: Theory and Practice*, 106–20. Belmont: Wadsworth, 1991.

Pierre, Jon. 'The Marketization of the State.' In Guy Peters and Donald Savoie, eds., *Governance in a Changing Environment*. Montreal: McGill-Queen's University Press, 1995.

Pierson, Paul. *Dismantling the Welfare State? Reagan, Thatcher and the Politics of Retrenchment*. Cambridge: Cambridge University Press, 1994.

Porter, John, *The Vertical Mosaic: An Analysis of Social Class and Power in Canada*. Toronto: University of Toronto Press, 1965.

Redden, Candace Johnson. 'Health Care as Citizenship Development: Revisioning Social Rights and Entitlement.' *Canadian Journal of Political Science*, March 2002.

– 'Rationing Care in the Community: Engaging Citizens in Health Care Decision Making.' *Journal of Health Politics, Policy and Law* 24/6 (December 1999), 1363–89.

– 'Through the Looking Glass: Federal Provincial Decision Making for Health Policy.' Institute of Intergovernmental Relations, Queen's University, Working Paper no. 6, 1998.

Rioux, Marcia. 'Appropriate Uses of Law in Health Policy: Three Views.' In Margaret A. Somerville, ed., *Do We Care? Renewing Canada's Commitment to Health*. Montreal: McGill-Queen's University Press, 1999.

Rousseau, Jean-Jacques. 'Letter to M. D'Alembert on the Theatre.' In Allan Bloom, trans., *Politics and the Arts*. New York: Free Press, 1960.

Saltman, Richard, and Josep Figueras. *European Health Care Reform: Analysis of Current Strategies*. Copenhagen: World Health Organization Regional Publications, European Series no. 72, 1997.

Sandel, Michael. *Democracy's Discontent: America in Search of a Public Philosophy*. Cambridge: Harvard University Press, 1996.

Sanders, Lynn. 'Against Deliberation.' *Political Theory* 25/3 (1997), 347–76.

Saskatchewan, HealNet: Health Services Utilization and Research Commission. *Regionalization at Age Five: Views of Saskatchewan Health Care Decision-Makers*. December 1997.

Saskatchewan, Saskatchewan Health, Policy and Planning Branch. *Interprovin-*

cial Comparisons: Provincial/ Territorial Health Services and Selected Data. February, 1998.

– *Annual Report 1996–1997*.

– *Health Renewal Is Working. Progress Report*. October 1996.

– *A Framework of Accountability. The Minister of Health and District Health Boards*. October 1995.

– *Supporting Wellness: Supportive Services in Saskatchewan. A Policy Framework*. March 1995.

– *Planning Guide for Saskatchewan Health Districts. Part III: Facilities Planning*. 1994.

– *Guidelines for Developing an Integrated Palliative Care Service*. April 1994.

– *Planning Guide for Saskatchewan Health Districts. Part II: Program Planning*. April 1994.

– *A Guide to Core Services for Saskatchewan Health Districts*. July 1993.

– *Planning Guide for Saskatchewan Health Districts*. March 1993.

– *User's Guide to the Health Districts Act*. March 1993.

– *Health Needs Assessment Guide for Saskatchewan Health Districts*. January 1993.

– *Health District Development Guide*. October 1992.

– *A Saskatchewan Vision for Health: A Framework for Change*. August 1992.

– *A Guide to Community Health Centres in Saskatchewan*.

Saskatchewan Association of Health Organizations (SAHO). *Health System Directions Part II: Objectives and Strategies*. July 1998.

– *Health System Directions Part I: Continuing the Vision*. March 1998.

Saul, John Ralston. 'Health Care at the End of the Twentieth Century: Confusing Symptoms for Systems.' In Margaret A. Somerville, ed., *Do We Care? Renewing Canada's Commitment to Health*. Montreal: McGill-Queen's University Press, 1999.

Schick, Allen. 'Budgetary Adaptations to Resource Scarcity.' In Charles Levine and Irene Rubin, eds., *Fiscal Stress and Public Policy*. London: Sage, 1980.

Schneider, Cathy Lisa. 'Racism, Drug Policy, and AIDS.' *Political Science Quarterly* 113/3, 1998, 427–46.

'75 Per Cent of Canadians in Favour of Health Care User Fees, Poll Finds.' *National Post*, 12 January 2000.

Shapiro, Ian. *The Evolution of Rights in Liberal Theory*. Cambridge: Cambridge University Press, 1986.

Shilts, Randy. *And The Band Played On: Politics, People, and the AIDS Epidemic*. New York: Penguin Books, 1987.

Simms, Maurice. 'Marketing Takes New Tacks.' *Globe and Mail*, 12 August 1997.

Smiley, Donald V., ed. *The Rowell-Sirois Report. An Abridgement of Book 1 of the*

Royal Commission on Dominion-Provincial Relations. Toronto: McClelland and Stewart, 1964.

Smith, Miriam. 'Retrenching the Sacred Trust: Medicare and Canadian Federalism.' In François Rocher and Miriam Smith, eds., *New Trends in Canadian Federalism*. Peterborough: Broadview Press, 1995.

Somerville, Margaret A., ed. *Do We Care? Renewing Canada's Commitment to Health*. Montreal: McGill-Queen's University Press, 1999.

Soss, Joe. 'Welfare Provision, Civil Society, and Democracy in the United States.' Paper prepared for The World Project on Civil Society Author's Conference, Center for the Study of Voluntary Organizations and Service, Washington, DC, 3–4 June 1999.

Sunstein, Cass. 'Beyond the Republican Revival.' *Yale Law Review*, 97 (1988), 1539–90.

Taylor, Charles. 'Multiculturalism and "the Politics of Recognition."' In Amy Gutmann, ed., *Multiculturalism: Examining the Politics of Recognition*, 25–73. Princeton: Princeton University Press, 1994.

Taylor, Malcolm. 'Health Insurance: The Roller-coaster in Federal-Provincial Relations.' In David Shugarman and Reg Whitaker, eds., *Federalism and Political Community*, 73–92. Peterborough: Broadview Press, 1989.

– *Health Insurance and Canadian Public Policy: The Seven Decisions That Created The Canadian Health Insurance System*. 2nd ed. Montreal: McGill-Queen's University Press, 1987.

– *Health Insurance and Canadian Public Policy: The Seven Decisions that Created the Canadian Health Insurance System*. 1st ed. Montreal and Kingston: McGill-Queen's University Press, 1978.

Taylor, Malcolm, H. Michael Stevenson, and A. Paul Williams. *Medical Perspectives on Canadian Medicare: Attitudes of Canadian Physicians to Policies and Problems of the Medical Care Insurance Program*. Toronto: York University, Institute for Behavioural Research, 1984.

Tindal, C. Richard, and Susan Nobes Tindal. *Local Government in Canada*. Toronto: McGraw-Hill Ryerson, 1995.

Tuck, Richard. *Natural Rights Theories: Their Origin and Development*. Cambridge: Cambridge University Press, 1979.

Tully, James. *Strange Multiplicity: Constitutionalism in an Age of Diversity*. Cambridge: Cambridge University Press, 1995.

Tuohy, Carolyn Hughes. *Accidental Logics: The Dynamics of Change in the Health Care Arena in the United States, Britain and Canada*. New York: Oxford University Press, 1999.

– 'Social Policy: Two Worlds.' In Michael Atkinson, ed., *Governing Canada: Institutions and Public Policy*. Toronto: Harcourt Brace Jovanovich, 1993.

- *Policy and Politics in Canada: Institutionalized Ambivalence.* Philadelphia: Temple University Press, 1992.
- 'Health Care in Canada.' In William M. Chandler and Christian W. Zollner, eds., *Challenges to Federalism: Policy-Making in Canada and the Federal Republic of Germany.* Kingston: Institute of Intergovernmental Relations, 1989.
- 'Medicine and the State in Canada: The Extra-Billing Issue in Perspective.' *Canadian Journal of Political Science* 21/2 (1988), 268–96.
- 'Conflict and Accommodation in the Canadian Health Care System.' In Robert Evans and G.L. Stoddart, eds., *Medicare at Maturity,* 393–434. Calgary: University of Calgary Press, 1986.
Turner, Bryan, ed. *Citizenship and Social Theory.* London: Sage, 1993.
UNAIDS. Joint United Nations Programme on HIV/AIDS. UNAIDS and the World Health Organization. *AIDS Epidemic Update.* Dec. 1999.
U.S. Department of Health and Human Services. Health Care Financing Administration. *Health Care Financing Review* 17 (Spring 1996).
Verghese, Abraham. *My Own Country: A Doctor's Story.* New York: Vintage Books, 1995.
Vickers, Jill. 'Why Should Women Care about Federalism?' In *Canada the State of the Federation.* Kingston: Institute of Intergovernmental Relations, Queen's University, 1995.
Waldman v Medical Services Commission of British Columbia. 30 July 1997. Supreme Court of British Columbia, Docket numbers A952722, A961607.
Watney, Simon. 'Practices of Freedom: "Citizenship" and the Politics of Identity in the Age of AIDS.' In Jonathan Rutherford, ed., *Identity: Community Culture Difference.* New York: New York University Press, 1990.
Whitaker, Reg. 'Rights in a Free and Democratic Society: Abortion.' In David Shugarman and Reg Whitaker, eds., *Federalism and Political Community.* Peterborough: Broadview, 1989.
White, Joseph. '(Almost) Nothing New under the Sun: Why the Work of Budgeting Remains Incremental.' In Naomi Caiden and Joseph White, eds., *Budgeting, Policy, Politics.* New Brunswick, NJ: Transaction Publishers, 1995.
Wilbur, J.R.H. *The Bennett New Deal: Fraud or Portent?* (Toronto: Copp Clark, 1968.
Wildavsky, Aaron, and Naomi Caiden. *The New Politics of the Budgetary Process.* New York: Longman, 1997.
Wilkinson, Richard G. 'The Epidemiological Transition: From Material Scarcity to Social Disadvantage.' *Daedalus,* Fall 1994, 61–78.
Wilson, James Q. *American Government: Institutions and Policies.* Toronto: D.C. Heath, 1992.

World Bank. *World Development Report: Knowledge for Development 1998/99.* New York: Oxford University Press, 1999.

– *Investing in Health.* New York: Oxford University Press, 1993.

World Health Organization. *Making a Difference.* Geneva: WHO: 1999.

Wrobel, Marion G. *The Federal Deficit and Universality of Social Programs.* Ottawa: Library of Parliament, Economics Division, 1989.

York, Geoffrey. *The High Price of Health: A Patient's Guide to the Hazards of Medical Politics.* Toronto: James Lorimer, 1987.

Young, Iris Marion. *Inclusion and Democracy.* Oxford: Oxford University Press, 2000.

– *Intersecting Voices: Dilemmas of Gender, Political Philosophy and Policy.* Princeton: Princeton University Press, 1997.

– *Justice and the Politics of Difference.* Princeton: Princeton University Press, 1990.

– 'Polity and Group Difference: A Critique of the Ideal of Universal Citizenship.' *Ethics* 99 (1989), 250–74.

Young, Robert. 'Dispensing With Moral Rights.' *Political Theory* 6 (1978), 63–74.

Index